DATE DUE

MR 17 '10			
APR 0 4 2012			
JUL 08 2013			
OCT 08 2013			
7/10/19 ILL			

Demco, Inc. 38-293

THE FAMILY THAT COULDN'T SLEEP

D. T. MAX

THE FAMILY THAT COULDN'T SLEEP

A Medical Mystery

RANDOM HOUSE | NEW YORK

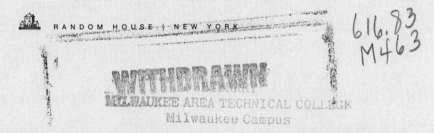

Published in the United States by Random House,
an imprint of The Random House Publishing Group,
a division of Random House, Inc., New York.

RANDOM HOUSE and colophon are registered
trademarks of Random House, Inc.

Portions of this book first appeared in The New York
Times Magazine *in 2001 and 2004.*

LIBRARY OF CONGRESS CATALOGING-IN-PUBLICATION DATA

Max, D. T. (Daniel T.)
    The family that couldn't sleep: a medical mystery/D. T. Max.—1st ed.
        p. cm.
    Includes index.
    ISBN: 1-4000-6245-4 (hardcover: alk. paper)
    1. Prion diseases.   2. Fatal familial insomnia.
3. Prions.   4. Sleep disorders.   I. Title.
RA644.P93M39 2006
616.8'3—dc22   2006043885

Printed in the United States of
America on acid-free paper

www.atrandom.com

9 8 7 6 5 4 3 2 1

FIRST EDITION

Book design by Barbara M. Bachman

For Sarah

Dove andrai tu andrò anch'io
e dove starai tu io pure starò

Now all my hours are trances;
And all my nightly dreams
Are where the dark eye glances,
And where thy footstep gleams,
In what ethereal dances,
By what Italian streams.

—EDGAR ALLAN POE, "The Assignation"

Protein, so far as we know, does not replicate itself all by itself, not on this planet anyway. Looked at this way, the [prion] seems the strangest thing in all biology and, until someone in some laboratory figures out what it is, a candidate for Modern Wonder.

—LEWIS THOMAS

CONTENTS

In October 1997, Stanley Prusiner, a professor at the University of California–San Francisco who had spent twenty-five years studying prions, went to Stockholm to receive the prize he called "the big one" from the King of Sweden. His great achievement was to show that the prion (pronounced "*pree*-on"), the infectious agent responsible for bovine spongiform encephalopathy, or mad cow disease, Creutzfeldt-Jakob disease, and a disease in sheep called scrapie, was not a virus or a bacterium but a protein, a nonliving thing. Protein, as the name suggests, is prime, proto matter. ("These agents," one prion researcher told a documentary film interviewer, "are almost immortal.")

The fifty-five-year-old Prusiner's discovery, the Swedish academy noted, introduced "a new biological principle of infection" into science. Over the years, Prusiner, an ambitious man, had developed a taste for good wine and food. Now the Swedish elite entertained him at their finest restaurants while the press pursued him for his photograph and his ideas. The moment was just as he'd always dreamed it would be. Asked by the newspapers what was left now that he had the top prize in science, he said his new goal would be to work towards "an effective therapy for prion diseases." In 1998, he told an Israeli newspaper he thought he'd have a cure in five years.

Three years later, in 2001, when a family in the Veneto, the Italian region of small towns and farms outside Venice, held its first family reunion, Prusiner's words were on their minds. Family reunions are rare in Italy, because they are unnecessary: Italian families already do everything together; you can't reunite something that never disperses. This family had a special reason for its gatherings, though—many of its members carry a gene for a dreadful disease. Of noble origin, the family counts doctors, engineers, industrial managers, and a well-respected academic among its number.

But this family is cursed. For at least two centuries, its members have suffered from an inherited prion disease called fatal familial insomnia that strikes them, usually in their fifties, killing by depriving them of sleep. FFI is an autosomal dominant mutation, which means that a child of a parent with FFI has a 50 percent chance of getting it, too. In the general population the chance of having FFI is one in 30 million; within the affected branches of this Italian family, it is one in two.

The symptoms of FFI are remarkable and grim. Typically, one day in middle age, the sufferer finds that he has begun to sweat. A look in the mirror will show that his pupils have shrunk to pinpricks and he is holding his head in an odd, stiff way. (I write "he" for clarity, though men and women are equally affected.) Constipation is common, the women suddenly enter menopause and the men become impotent. The sufferer begins to have trouble sleeping and tries compensating with a nap in the afternoon, but to no avail. His blood pressure and pulse have become elevated and his body is in overdrive. Over the ensuing months, he tries desperately to sleep, sometimes closing his eyes but never succeeding in falling into more than a light stupor. FFI sufferers are sometimes able to enter a half sleep that is like a parody of the agitated dream sleep some people experience just before waking, but they can't go deeper to get real rest. Their exhaustion is immense, beyond comprehension.

Once the sufferer can no longer sleep, a downward progression ensues, as he loses his ability to walk or balance. Perhaps most tragic, the ability to think remains intact; sufferers know what is happening. At first, they can talk about it and even write down their thoughts. After a few more months, some lose this level of functioning. Once their bodies shut down, only the desperate look in their eyes shows that they know what is going on. But others can talk and reason until the end. In the terminal phase, usually about fifteen months after the disease has begun, they fall into a state of exhaustion resembling a coma and die. "When I began this work," Pierluigi Gambetti, the director of the national prion surveillance center at Case Western Reserve University School of Medicine in Cleveland, one of the discoverers of the disease, told me, "I used to think Alzheimer's was the worst disease you could get. But to see a loved one disintegrate in front of your eyes—and for that person to know it is happening? Somehow, the fact that it is so rare makes it even worse, it seems to me. I think now even a car accident would be less cruel."

This Italian family is one of a handful of families in the world afflicted with fatal familial insomnia. They can trace their disease back to the mid-eighteenth century, possibly to a Venetian doctor who lived near the Jewish ghetto, and with certainty from him to an aristocrat in the Veneto named Giuseppe and down to Vincenzo in the 1880s, Giovanni in the 1910s, Pietro in the 1940s, Assunta, Pierina, and Silvano in the last three decades of the twentieth century and on to . . . to whom? That question hangs over the group at its annual reunions.

In a sense, the answer is known. In the early 1990s, the University of Bologna, whose neurological institute specializes in sleep, tested many of the members of the family for the genetic mutation that causes FFI and has the results in its files. So who will die is known, although in what order family members will perish is not. And that someone will die soon is all but certain—at least thirty members of the family have died from FFI in the last century, fourteen since 1973, seven in the past decade. Among living family members, the laws of probability suggest that at least a dozen more carry the mutation that causes the disease.

Many lethal genetic diseases disappear on their own, because they bring about death before the carriers of the mutation can reproduce, but not FFI—at least not in this family. Because the disease usually strikes its sufferers after their childbearing years, and because most members of this family still decide to have children, FFI will live on through them. The decision to bring a child into the world who may die a horrible death in middle age is a difficult one. Bologna weighed this equation at the time it conducted its genetic tests and decided it would not inform the members of family whether they had the mutation or not so they could not use the information in making reproductive decisions. The family gave its consent to being kept ignorant, and to my knowledge no family member has terminated a pregnancy out of fear of passing the syndrome on.

Bologna framed the family's problem, but it did not solve it. Family members still must wait for the tautly held head and pinpoint pupils that are the first sign of the disease, then the sweating and shivering that follow, the handkerchief always on the brow or the shirt that has to be changed at midday or the sudden menopause, and the awful next step, when the sufferer begins not to sleep.

Sleep is central to us. It's central to the experience of being human. That every person goes to sleep every night, that we all seek a warm, safe place to cover and restore ourselves for a third of every day, that people of every race and every age do this, that we have done it since before we were *Homo sapiens,* is amazing. Lying down to sleep is the most childlike of gestures, the most trusting. It is at the same time a symbol of ebbing life force, a rehearsal for the day we will lie down and not get up.

Sleep is homeostatic—that is, it is controlled by the body's internal balance. When we have slept enough, our body wakes us up, and when we have not slept enough, it forces us to sleep, a soft unyielding power pushing us down. When you stay awake too long, you experience a mussy-headedness, a feeling of going under. Even as you force your eyes to stay open, sleep is flowing in through your ears and nose and mouth, rising around your legs and arms, weighing down your head until your chin drops to your chest. But the feeling that sleep comes and conquers us is an illusion; sleep is always in us. It is something we are born knowing how to do. Actually, we sleep even before that, in utero. By the third month in the womb our lives are defined by sleeping and waking. One of the first things the brain learns is to turn the body off.

That sleep is one of the body's most primal functions makes the fact that we don't really know its biological purpose even stranger. Did it once exist to keep us out of harm's way for part of the day—to make us lie low while predators were hunting? Is it time reserved for the central processing unit that is the brain to devote to updating its databases? Or perhaps the unconsciousness of sleep is exactly its purpose: sleep exists to help us forget useless information. Because everyone feels better after a good night's sleep, it's natural to believe that sleep makes us healthier—by improving immune function, repairing damaged tissue, improving nerve connections. The early-seventeenth-century writer Richard Burton catalogued its virtues in *The Anatomy of Melancholy*. Sleep, he wrote, "moystens and fattens the body, concocts, and helpes digestion . . . expels cares, pacifies the mind, refresheth the weary limbs after long work." No doubt sleep does this and more, but that does not explain its existence, as studies have shown that lying quietly awake achieves all these ends better. Still, we sleep because we, and every other animal, must. "If sleep does not serve an absolutely vital function, it is the greatest mistake that evolution ever made," the American sleep researcher Allan Rechtschaffen once said.

Humans, being human, have tried to unmake that mistake—as night watchmen, truck drivers, astronauts. The modern record for voluntary sleeplessness is held by an American teenager, Randy Gardner. In a competition for the science prize at his high school, Gardner stayed awake for eleven days on doughnuts, pinball, and TV in 1964. "Then I went to sleep for about fourteen hours," he said. "When I woke up, I felt like a million bucks. Like I'd just been born." The next night he slept normally.

Most of us, though, would collapse after three days of sleeplessness. Before collapsing, we would show some symptoms similar to those of the FFI family. We would sweat. We would be confused. We would grow clumsy. If we went without sleep for much longer, we would begin to hallucinate and lose touch with reality. But blessedly, for the more than 99.999 percent of us who do not suffer from FFI, homeostasis eventually would reassert itself: we would fall asleep, and with only a few hours of slumber, be sane again. With a few hours more, our bodies and minds would be completely repaired. The rebound would be remarkable—like Randy Gardner's rebirth.

During the epidemic of Von Economo's disease, or encephalitis lethargica, in Europe and America during the second and third decades of the twentieth century, millions suffered from hypersomnolence, an inability to wake up. But there were also a small number of cases, mostly in Italy as it happens, of people who couldn't sleep, the closest parallel to the symptoms of FFI that we know of. Among these, some were intensely active, twitching, jerking, and racing around their hospital wards with pointless exuberance until their deaths, presumably from exhaustion. But others had a lower-key chronic insomnia—not a mania but an ongoing state of agitation and neurosis. Their condition would not seem life-threatening—and yet they too died. What did they die from? No experiment has ever answered that question. Allan Rechtschaffen came close by keeping rats awake until they died, at around fourteen days. During this time, the rats overproduced adrenalinelike hormones, in effect going into overdrive, and underproduced thyroid hormones, used by the body for weight and temperature control. They ate aggressively but kept losing weight and their skin began to break down. Eventually, they began to shiver and they died. Clearly, something had gone wrong with their internal regulatory functioning—their autonomic nervous system—but on autopsy, nothing sufficient to explain their deaths was found. It is almost as if a tautology had killed them: if you force a rat to stay awake, it dies from lack of sleep.

Rechtschaffen's experiment is not a pleasant one to contemplate. To watch any animal endure insomnia is uncomfortable; to watch a human suffer from it is horrifying. Many in the Italian family have had this experience. They have watched sleep begin to evade a loved one and then taken him or her to the doctor, who, bewildered, sent the family to a specialist, who, being a specialist, made a diagnosis. It was always the wrong diagnosis: encephalitis, a swelling of the brain, meningitis, anxiety, depression, schizophrenia, or, in fact, Von Economo's disease. John Wilesmith, the British epidemiologist who in the late 1980s traced the cause of mad cow disease, which is closely related to FFI, to contaminated feed, told me that "drunken cow" would have been a better name for the disease he studied. The sickness that afflicts the FFI family is also often taken for drunkenness. Doctors usually presume that the sufferers are alcoholic, until they can prove otherwise.

Amid all this suffering, the family can only do what it has always done: take herbs, pray to God, and avoid stress, which family lore— and recent scientific studies—says brings FFI on. "My family believed that the best way to prevent the disease was not to mention it," explained one relative, whose father had died from FFI just three months before the family's first reunion.

I attended that reunion in July 2001. It was meant to mark a break with the family's historical attitude of helplessness with regard to their disease, and to come up with a strategy for pursuing a cure. Gathered were about fifty family members, at once embarrassed, nervous, hopeful, and driven against their native caution to participate. In attending the meeting, they were admitting that the family had a problem, and that a concerted effort might find a solution.

It was a sunny day, and the flowers were in bloom along the roads and canals of the Veneto. Sheep and cows grazed in the nearby fields and locals bicycled back and forth from the markets, ducking around the traffic barriers at the train crossing. Family members had come from as far away as Padua, which though only an hour by car, represented a considerable journey: Italians like to remain *in paese,* close to home.

Now they gathered in the house of a family member who has lost an uncle, two aunts, and a grandfather to the disease. The man owns a small business. He makes good money and he built a new ranch-style house whose spacious central hall would not be out of place in northern California or the Hamptons. The light pours into his house. He does not worry or think much about the disease, unlike his sister Elisabetta. This is common among families with genetic diseases: members tend to divide between the ignorers and the burden carriers. In this family, Lisi, as the family calls Elisabetta, is a burden carrier. Before the meeting she took me on a bike ride down the cypress-lined lane to the town cemetery, where many of her relatives are buried. We looked at the pictures of her uncle and her grandfather and she seemed on the verge of tears.

Lisi and her husband, Ignazio, a doctor of internal medicine, were crucial in the discovery of the disease. Ignazio was the first doctor to pay attention to what was going on. Instead of throwing up his hands, as generations of medical practitioners had done before him, he embraced the mystery, digging through records of the spectacular and confusing symptoms to get to the neurological alterations that were bringing about the deaths in his wife's family. Meanwhile, Lisi, herself trained as a nurse, was on the telephone with her relatives, extracting information that they had left unexamined during two centuries of fear and humiliation. What did Rita die of? What about Maria? The doctors said schizophrenia but on the death certificate they put meningitis? What had the family believed? Did any of the siblings also behave oddly?

Shame led the different branches of the family to withdraw from one another over the centuries. Lisi reversed that isolation. She is small and intense, with blond-brown hair and bags under her eyes: she never sleeps well. "Is there a pill that makes you forget?" she asked me once. Sometimes she trembles when she speaks. She doesn't drive, getting around her little town with its disused canals by bicycle. Ignazio once got out a book and showed me a picture of Albrecht Dürer's famous drawing of melancholy. "*Ecco Lisi,*" he said. This is Lisi.

Ignazio led the meeting. In his early fifties then, with gray hair, soft eyes, and the bowed mustache of a leading man in an operetta, he exuded patience. Over the years, his work—he is now head of internal medicine at Treviso's hospital—gave him a good bedside manner. He speaks slowly when he speaks about disease, curbing his intense intelligence, always aware that the mind resists the idea of sickness in the body. While he has seen the misery FFI brings, as a doctor Ignazio can also admire its work—the extraordinary way Stanley Prusiner's Nobel-honored prions hollow out the thalamus, the part of the brain that is destroyed by FFI, and how unusual this pathology is. Having also helped define a new disease, Ignazio has a sense of ownership (alongside horror at what FFI has done to the family he married into), an understandable need to defend his claim before the big-name researchers—the Prusiners of the world—who, with their multimillion-dollar grants and press officers, are always eroding the credit he deserves.

I sat next to Ignazio that day, the two of us behind a child's school desk, and looked out across the terra-cotta floor at the family seated in a circle around us. I was there as a visitor, a guest, a journalist who had written about the family, and an American, from the land where technology fixes everything. Ignazio welcomed the group, told them how important this meeting could prove for the future of the family and added that at that moment, fortunately, no one was dying of the disease. "I hope this never changes," he added, "but . . ." He spread out his hands as if to say, We all know what hope is worth.

Everyone acknowledged this truth but no one cried—if anyone in the room was thinking about death, they were also taking comfort in how far in the future it seemed. Mostly, they were here to see where they stood and to see that others stood with them. There were almost no elder members there, which I assumed was the result of a combination of the toll the disease took and, among those still living, the knowledge that they were old enough to be free from risk, but it turned out more to have to do with culture and shame. When Italians think someone is being unnecessarily brusque or aggressive, they say he is being *"anglosassone,"* Anglo-Saxon. The idea of this first reunion was very *anglosassone,* spurred by the success that AIDS activists had had in getting resources devoted to a treatment for their disease. Identify yourselves, join forces, approach sympathizers, push your government, and get what you want. That was not the Italian way. Who could blame the elderly for staying away from this meeting? They did not grow up in a place where disability and disease found much cultural support.

Then Ignazio explained what a prion disease was: a sickness caused by a protein that becomes deformed. In the case of FFI this deformation usually begins when a person reaches his or her fifties. It was the first time many of the family members had heard anything about their family illness, beyond that it was inherited. Ignazio added that the family was once the only family in the world known to have the mutation, but that there were now other families—not many, but around forty, spread around the world. This confused many of the audience. "I don't understand," one family member objected, "how we can be related to a bunch of Japanese."

Ignazio steadily explained that the two families weren't related: the same mutation can occur in different families in different places at different times. He went on to explain that prion researchers, including Prusiner himself, also hoped FFI might shed light on a range of diseases that have always eluded medical understanding, among them Parkinson's, Huntington's, amyotrophic lateral sclerosis (Lou Gehrig's disease), and Alzheimer's disease. These were not prion diseases, he said, but diseases in which other proteins also grew deformed. The applicability of FFI to other protein diseases, along with the spread of mad cow disease, was why the family's situation was not as hopeless as it seemed, he pointed out. They could be of use to others.

If something about FFI could prove useful to millions of others, then maybe a cure really was at hand. The group suddenly seemed more animated. "Why didn't we do this sooner?" asked one young family member, who previously had been known to block any initiative around the disease. Soon, other young members of the group were asking about a cure. Ignazio was cautious. "Work toward a cure is going on," he said, "but the disease is difficult." Publicity, he added, would speed things up.

That was where I came in. Until recently the family members had all kept silent, even to one another. They saw isolation and denial as self-protection. And some people at the reunion regarded me warily. "Why are you here?" one of the young men asked me. Yes, I was going to write about them, I explained, but I also had a disease. It was not fatal and not a prion disease, but, like prion diseases and neurodegenerative diseases, mine involved the failure of the body's proteins to fold properly. As it progressed, my disease, which had never been satisfactorily identified, caused my legs and my arms to weaken. I already wore braces on my legs. Though the two diseases were related only because protein misformation underlay both of them—mine was not a prion disease; theirs was not a neuromuscular disease—a cure for theirs might lead to a cure for mine or vice versa.

Some of the people in the circle nodded, some kept silent, but one young man, whose mother had died of FFI when he was a child, did not think this made my presence acceptable. He understood the unbridgeable distance between what he might have and what I had. "*Sei un curioso,*" he said: You're an onlooker, a gawker.

The family had attracted gawkers before, and the experience had been scarring. The story of a relative named Silvano—Lisi's uncle, a debonair executive who died of FFI in 1984—found its way into the Italian papers after Pierluigi Gambetti and others published a report on the disease in the *New England Journal of Medicine* in 1986. "Help us, we're dying of insomnia" ran a typical headline in an Italian newspaper. After such articles, children in the neighborhood of the Veneto where Ignazio and Lisi live came by their house at night, mooing, pretending they were mad cows. Such cruelty left its mark on the family.

I told the group that the chief goal of my book would be to remind the reader that we are all mortal and must live with the awareness of our own mortality, that though death may come to their family in one particularly horrid form, none of us is exempt. We all die, at once, good and bad deaths. Everyone in the room acknowledged the truth of that, Italy being if no longer a religious country, still a soulful one.

America had a good reputation in Italy, and it helped that I was American (this was before the invasion of Iraq). They asked me for my opinion on how to combat their disease, and I suggested a foundation to raise research funds, an idea which Ignazio seconded, and the group liked. Yes, of course: a foundation would raise money to cure the disease. Why hadn't they thought of that before? Ignazio had a friend who could design a website; one young man suggested its symbol be a man yawning, and everyone laughed. The family went back out into the sunshine, full of enthusiasm, ready for a new chapter. This was the modern era of cures and they were going to be part of it. Write quickly, one said to me.

This is a book about prion diseases—what they are, what causes them, who they afflict, how we might cure them, and how we found out what we know about them. Because prion diseases come from three sources—some are caused by inheritance, like FFI, some by chance, like one form of Creutzfeldt-Jakob disease, others by human intervention, like mad cow disease—our relationship to prion disease is a microcosm of our relationship to illness in general. Sometimes illness strikes us—a gene goes wrong, a cell multiplies out of control—and some times we bring it on ourselves—we poison our environment; we taint our food; we force pathogens out of their natural habitat and into ours. Against random disease, we strive relentlessly; against diseases we bring about, we are sometimes humbled, but in the end we try to invent our way out of that problem too.

Prion diseases are a fascinating medical mystery, because they appear to be the only disease that takes those three forms: genetic, infectious, and accidental (often called "sporadic"). The theory of prion diseases—I write "theory" because the gold standard of proof has not yet been met—is that prions can perform this triple trick because they are agents unique in biology: infectious proteins. That is, they are proteins that behave like viruses or bacteria.

Until the discovery of prions, scientists thought proteins could not have this ability. They knew them as the building blocks of the body— "nature's robots," in the dismissive words of one book on them— things the body made and, when their function was fulfilled, disposed of. The human body has roughly a hundred thousand different proteins. Hair and muscle are mostly protein; skin is made up of proteins too. There are also tens of thousands more proteins within the cell about which we know little or nothing, the functioning of the various proteins in the body being the last great frontier of human biology. A recent proteomics conference title caught this sense of challenge: "Human Proteome Project: 'Genes Were Easy.' "

Certainly easier than prions. We don't even know what prions do when healthy—they may possibly aid in memory; in yeast, they have been shown to make genetic adaptation easier. Because they can be found in all mammals, it is safe to assume that they have a function—otherwise the gene responsible for them would have dropped out or become inoperative somewhere along the course of animal evolution.

How do prions infect their victims? The body manufactures proteins as ribbons, which then fold into three-dimensional shapes that allow them to fulfill whatever function they have. Most proteins, because of the arrangement of their atoms, have only one such shape, but prion proteins—the theory goes—have two, one normal, the second infectious and lethal.

Once the first abnormal prion appears, it begins to spread in the body through a process called "conformational influence"—"conformation" meaning "shape." After one prion becomes malignant, the way it's folded allows it to bond with adjoining healthy prion proteins, and the bonding causes these prion proteins in turn to fold wrongly and bond with others, making them fold wrongly, too. The chain reaction extends from protein to protein, normal prion protein changing to lethal prion in a series of Jekyll-to-Hyde conversions. Cells that have the misformed prions in them sicken and die, for reasons we don't really understand, but the effect of all these misfolded proteins on the delicate cells of the sufferer's brain is overwhelming: the brain tissue of prion disease victims is full of gaps, areas where all the cells have died, as if an explosion had gone off. Writing of her father, who had died of Creutzfeldt-Jakob disease, one woman posted on an e-mail list: "My husband seen his brain X-ray and said it looked like someone shot him with a .22 shotgun."

—

For biologists the prion theory is a heresy. To them, the word "infection" means something specific—a disease process brought about by living things, more exactly by things with nucleic acids or genetic material in them. Whatever else proteins are, they are not living and have no nucleic acid. The theory of prions thus threatens to unmake the defining moment in biology. In 1862, Louis Pasteur boiled broth to kill the microscopic life in it, put some of the liquid in a goose-necked flask, and showed that if nothing living ever reached the liquid, no life would ever grow there. The experiment had enormous practical impact; it gave doctors the knowledge they still use to save lives by showing that because infections were living, reproducing things, if you could keep an environment sterile, you could keep a patient healthy. Had infectious prions been in Pasteur's flask, curative medicine would never have gotten started. Doctors would still be competing with shamans and medicasters.

Because the possibility that infectious agents don't have to be alive violates a paradigm, various prion diseases have been around for a long time without anyone successfully connecting them. All that doctors and scientists knew before the current effort to find the underlying unifying principle began was what they could see: that there existed a small group of diseases with roughly similar symptoms, including loss of coordination and dementia, and with a perplexing absence of fever—one expects to see fever in an infection but in prion diseases one doesn't. Scientists also saw how these diseases had a tendency to burst into sudden outbreaks and then disappear, but they did not know why. The fact that the diseases had this ability, though, always lent urgency to the attempt to understand what was going on.

Prion diseases always seemed a threat, a threat whose urgency increased enormously when researchers discovered in the mid-1990s that a prion disease in cattle—specifically, bovine spongiform encephalopathy, or mad cow disease—could jump the species barrier and infect humans. The more scientists understood about prion diseases, the more it seemed possible that one misfolded protein could, in any living being, start a rapid process of misfolding and infection that would kill that individual and make its invisible way from one body to another and from one species to another. The fear of the potency of prions can be seen in the caution coroners and undertakers use in handling the bodies of prion disease victims. They bury them in nine-foot-deep graves. They warn the bereaved not to touch their dead. Sometimes they don't even allow their relatives in the same room as the closed casket. "The coroner here would not even let us have my husband's body," one woman wrote on a website for the relatives of prion disease sufferers. "We just had to have a memorial service."

It is enormously difficult to disinfect a prion. What kills viruses and bacteria barely affects them. Boiling will not disinfect them, nor will heat. You can't reliably "kill" a prion with radiation. You can't pour formaldehyde on it to render it harmless—in fact formaldehyde makes prions tougher. Not all bleaches can kill prions and those that can need to be highly concentrated. Prions bond to metal. They can be spread, for instance, when doctors reuse the electrodes planted in patients' brains for EEGs or by dental equipment. To be on the safe side now, some hospitals discard the tools they use to operate on or autopsy those with CJD after a single use. Prions endure in soil too. After a flock of sheep in Iceland came down with scrapie, they were killed, and the land left unoccupied for ten years. At that point, farmers brought in a new flock, which picked up the disease. Researchers once opened up a container with the preserved brain of a person who had died of a prion disease twenty years earlier and injected the tissue into lab animals. The animals contracted the disease.

Mad cow disease became the prion poster disease—gothic in its symptoms, its arrival as unexpected as its future was unpredictable, its spread in cattle the first prion outbreak witnessed in the modern era of molecular medicine, and its expansion into humans the first proven case of a prion disease jumping from one species to another. Mad cow has so far killed more than 150 people in Europe and threatens to spread to America. In fact, many think the disease may be here—either having arrived through contaminated beef or because it was already present in the form of chronic wasting disease, a native prion disease that affects deer and elk. According to these people, the only reason we don't know that Americans are dying of mad cow is either governmental incompetence or a deliberate cover-up. "If," one poster wrote in a 2006 New Year's message on a CJD website, "there was only some way to bring certain government agents and agencies, certain meat industry officials and politicians up on murder and attempted murder charges for intentionally misrepresenting the CJD plague. . . ."

Despite the trauma and fear chronicled in these pages, this book is meant to be, if not a tribute, at least an admiring acknowledgment of human achievement. Prions and the diseases they cause could not have been discovered by the research methods that so often dominate modern science. It required remarkable men and women making great imaginative leaps to build the theory of prion diseases. Two of these scientists—Carleton Gajdusek, who studied a tribe in Papua New Guinea afflicted with a prion disease called kuru that nearly exterminated them—and Stanley Prusiner at UC–San Francisco, who helped identify the key protein and then named it—won Nobel Prizes for their efforts. This book cannot do other than to admire their work and what it suggests about human potential, the interrogative, investigative, imaginative impulse that has made *Homo sapiens* the dominant animal on the planet.

But a surprising, second lesson prion diseases teach us is that the very thing that makes us who we are, our ambition, has laid us open to prion disease—not inherited kinds, such as fatal familial insomnia, but infectious kinds, such as mad cow disease. It now appears that certain types of breeding and feeding may have caused the great prion outbreaks, including scrapie in the eighteenth century, and mad cow and chronic wasting disease in our own times (and even a prion epidemic in prehistoric times). So this is also a book about a dangerous part of human nature that always accompanies the need to know, the need to remake. During the Renaissance, the Florentine humanist Pico della Mirandola defined man as *"plasteis et fictor,"* maker and molder of himself. But for humans that was never sufficient. They would be not just makers and molders of themselves. They would be makers and molders of the world around them. Humans had, as the Bible promised, dominion. It would be foolish not to exercise it.

This is not the first time our ambition has cost us as a species, either. Around ten thousand years ago, our ancestors began to farm. The motive to settle down and till the land was obvious. Farming provided a more stable food supply than hunting and foraging; it allowed humans to populate the earth more densely. But the decision to stay in one place also brought us into contact with bacteria and viruses that we barely knew before: measles, smallpox, and tuberculosis—diseases we caught from the animals we domesticated and only, finally, brought under control in the late nineteenth century, after they killed hundreds of millions of humans.

The prion story differs from the bacteria/virus story of early agricultural settlements in an interesting way too—it refutes the theory best laid out by Darwin that life consists of competition among individuals to propagate their genes. Prions are just proteins; they are not alive. They have no DNA to pass on. They are not in a competition with us, trying to increase their numbers, as viruses and bacteria are—they are just molecules, attracting and repelling and folding and misfolding according to chemical forces. The assumption that infectious diseases must embody a Darwinian struggle between attacker and defender made it hard for researchers to consider what other factors might play a significant role in sickness.

The competitive paradigm never did a very good job explaining diseases like FFI or CJD, let alone Alzheimer's or Parkinson's disease, in which the body also seems to damage itself by manufacturing defective proteins. Now we are much closer to knowing why: Parkinson's and Alzheimer's and many other neurodegenerative and neuromuscular diseases are not the result of conventional infections or immune system responses but a form of protein misfolding akin to prion diseases.

The discoveries in the field of prion diseases helped shed light on these conditions and may in time help to provide a cure. This coming extension of prions and the prion paradigm to other protein diseases, I believe, is but the first application we will find for them—there will be others, some biological, some not. We will continue finding uses for prions because we did so much to make them happen, and with their aimlessness and their casual ability to inflict damage they fit our postmodern mindset well. For symbolic as much as environmental reasons, we are in the era of the prion and can be in no other. Prions sit at the intersection of humans' ambition and nature's unpredictability, and it is hard to say which is more dangerous.

PART 1

ALONE IN THE NIGHT

CHAPTER 1

THE DOCTORS' DILEMMA VENICE, *1765*

*Who is it that says there is a great difference between a good physician
and a bad one; yet very little between a good one and none at all?*

—ARTHUR YOUNG, Travels in Italy and France

In November 1765 a respected doctor from a good Venetian
family died in the Campo Santi Apostoli, near the Jewish ghetto in
Venice. The cause of his death was "an organic defect of the heart's
sack"—or so contemporary parish records state. In truth no one
would have known for sure what he suffered from and we can't know either. But priests ordinarily only wrote detailed descriptions of diseases
when what they saw was noteworthy, and it is intriguing that the de-
scription of the doctor's illness in the parish book is one of the longest
of the year.

The entry records that the deceased suffered for more than a year
from "intermittent difficulty in breathing" and adds that he was
bedridden and "totally paralyzed for two months" before his death.

Many of the doctor's descendants would experience similar symptoms in the course of dying from fatal familial insomnia, suggesting that the Venetian doctor may have been the earliest recorded case of a disease that has gone on to torment his relatives for more than two centuries.

Mid-eighteenth-century Venice was a place of gaiety and vice. The city always had a fairy-tale aspect, but until the seventeenth century its irreality was checked by an appetite for business. Venice stood at the crossroads of east and west, Asia and Europe, and it avidly cashed in on its location. But with the colonization of the Americas, trade turned the other way—across the Atlantic—and Venice began spending down its inheritance. Goethe, visiting the city in 1786, noted that the Venetians' lagoon was silting up, their trade "declining, their political power dwindling . . . Venice, like everything else that has a phenomenal existence, is subject to Time." The end was near, and everyone there knew it.

Venice's fall, though, was the time of its greatest opulence. This was the era of Casanova's wanton memoirs and the splendid Venetian regattas and processions painted by Canaletto and Francesco Guardi. One story may help to convey the moment: in 1709, there was a ball at the home of a Venetian noble in honor of the king of Denmark, Frederick IV. As the king danced with one of the guests, a newly married noblewoman named Caterina Quirini, his buckle caught a string of pearls that adorned the belt of her dress, scattering them on the floor. The lady paid them no mind. The king was about to bend down to retrieve the pearls, whereupon her husband stood up, walked across the dance floor, and crushed them under his feet, while his wife danced on.

Venice was a hereditary oligarchy. Its ruling class—its doges, procurators, and ambassadors—were drawn from two hundred families whose names, like that of the Quirini, had been inscribed in a "book of nobility" in the early fourteenth century. The Venetian doctor descended from one of these patrician families, great merchants and secretaries of state, whose surname adorned one of the central squares of the city. Though he was not himself entitled to wear the red toga that indicated patrician status, he enjoyed many of the other privileges of high birth in the republic.

The doctor had a three-story palazzo on a canal and a country home in the Veneto (both still standing today). The country house was in a town near the Piave River, a trip the doctor could make in three days, by crossing the lagoon by gondola to Portegrandi and then continuing in a carriage. In the country, on terra firma, a doctor of good family could play cards and chess with well-born friends, and supervise his gardens and the collection of rents from his tenant farmers, all the while staying clear of the infections summer brought to Venice.

If the doctor did have fatal familial insomnia—the idea has been suggested by his descendants in their search for the origin of their mutation—he likely would have noticed his first symptoms there in the summer of 1764. His servants, seeing his glassy eyes and sweaty forehead, might have gossiped that a witch had hexed him, but the doctor would not have entertained that idea for a moment. He was a graduate of the School of Medicine at Padua, the best in Europe. For him, sickness was not a magical but a natural process. The scientific method was blossoming in the Venetian state, of which Padua was a part. Its secular saint, Galileo, had set out the goal for all to see. "Science," he had written, could be found "in a huge book that stands always open before our eyes—I mean the universe." To read it, though, you needed to understand the language it was written in: "the language is mathematics." A physician's job, then, was to substitute exact observation for speculation, to look with vision unclouded by metaphysics or theology.

The sleepless doctor could trace his medical pedigree directly to Galileo. Galileo had taught the monk Castell, who had taught Borelli, who had taught the anatomist Malpighi, who had taught Valsalva, who had taught Morgagni, who had taught him. They had many of them learned their craft in the Acquapendente in Padua, the most beautiful autopsy theater in Europe. Its wooden balconies rose up in a narrowing series of concentric ovals—a "high funnel," as Goethe described it—from which the audience could look down on the human body lying in Euclidean splendor. Italian doctors were brilliant with their scalpels; seen from above, their work would have seemed to promise to the eager medical student the doctor had once been that if you studied nature hard enough, it would give up its secrets.

That promise wasn't working for him now, though. He was no longer sleeping well and he did not know why. In the beginning, the feeling might not have been unpleasant—he could stay up all night playing cards or maybe read Morgagni's famous comparisons of the body to a machine, published just a few years before. Just as any machine needed rest to prepare for the next day, so did the human. Yet the doctor's machinery seemed to be running nonstop. He was sweating more and more and his servants would by now be bringing him fresh shirts several times a day.

If the doctor had turned to contemporary authorities on insomnia, he would have found little of use. Sleep, even now a mystery in many ways to science and medicine, was utterly obscure to the doctors of his time, who were still struggling to understand what went on in plain sight in the day. Indeed, the unsleeping doctor would have had to go all the way back to Galen, the ancient Roman physician whose teachings had dominated medicine until Galileo had challenged him a century before. Galen had learned most of what *he* knew about sleep from Aristotle, who had pronounced confidently on the question (as he had on most scientific issues). "All things that have a natural function," he wrote authoritatively in *On Sleep and Dreams,* "must, whenever they exceed the time for which they can do a certain thing, lose their capacity and cease from doing it, e.g., the eyes from seeing. Necessarily, everything that wakes must be capable of sleeping. For it is unable to be active at all times." Aristotle proposed that sleep was a byproduct of eating. After a person had a big meal the warm fumes from the process of digestion entered the veins, thence to the brain, and thither to the heart, the seat of consciousness, where their cooling brought about sleep. Galen, writing five centuries after him, corrected Aristotle— the warm meal went directly to the brain, where it plugged the pores by which sensations entered and exited.

It is unlikely the Venetian doctor took either Galen or Aristotle seriously. Both would have seemed speculative to him when compared to the certainties of the Acquapendente. Still, back in Venice now, to be on the safe side, he might have ordered his cook to produce bigger meals—roast fowls and hams and sausages and fish from the Adriatic doused in the heavy French sauces that were newly in style. If so, the results would have confirmed his skepticism about the learnedness of anyone who had not gone to Padua. He would have sat awake in a chair, his stomach distended, waiting for the meal to warm his head. To help the process along he would have had plenty of wine, as well—wine was particularly recommended for insomnia—and then sat up through the night until the sun rose over the Lido.

Or maybe he got up and went out, frustrated by the noise—the hawkers and prostitutes and gondoliers singing to one another filled the nighttime air of a city in which, as the fussy Goethe noted, "the people . . . appreciate volume more than anything else." If it was Lent, the doctor could have gone to one of the huge *carnevale* masked balls in the palaces on the Grand Canal, where, as a man of noble birth, he was always welcome. There, dressed as the *medico della peste,* he could have kept his vigil. It was the sort of wit Venetians admired—a doctor in the black cape, the long white nose, and the face mask of the plague fighter. Dressed this way, the only evidence of his problem would have been the twin pinpricks of his eyes, peering from behind his mask. He'd have come home to the sound of the Marangona, the great bell in Piazza San Marco, tolling the beginning of the work day, sleep still well beyond his grasp.

The doctor would have asked himself whether he had caught something. Infection was on the mind of mid-eighteenth-century Venice. The city had a public health department well versed in the subject. They burned the bedding of disease victims and left their clothes out in the sun and air for a week to help neutralize the contagion. But what were they neutralizing? Here there was less agreement. The predominant view was that infection was an invisible substance carried in the air as smell. Thus the plague doctor costume of *carnevale* had a sponge at the tip of the long white nose, and workers who disinfected clothing for the Venetian authorities were also required to perfume the room and the personal effects of the deceased.

But in the lexicon of disease there was no infection that corresponded to what the doctor was feeling. He was not just hot but extraordinarily anxious, like a horse at full gallop, sweaty and prone to a shaking that seemed to come from deep within. He was exhausted, falling in and out of a light, dream-wracked sleep. His servants might have heard him knocking on his own window, thinking it was a door, or spied him preparing the leeches for use, swishing around imaginary water in the dark glass jar where he kept them. The servants would have gone into his room to waken him, followed by his distraught wife. He would not remember sleeping, nor would he feel at all rested. "I'm tired"—"*Mi so straco,*" he would say in Venetian. And when the servants had left the room, to his wife alone he would express his deepest horror: "*Mi divento mato.*" Was he indeed going crazy? Was he destined for the ships of fools, those boats in the farthest parts of the lagoon where the Serenissima housed the poor souls from whom God had taken the power of reason?

By now, he would also have consulted with the experts at Venice's collegium, the learned medical society. Unfortunately, his fellow practitioners had much the same knowledge he had: they knew the structures of the body, what the major organs did, and what they looked like when examined after death. But they really knew nothing about disease in the living. Still, then (as now) doctors believed in their own judgment, in knowing when to bleed and when to salve, when to prescribe cold baths and when to recommend warm wine. They would have focused on the fact that the doctor was sweating all the time. They might have taken his temperature—the thermometer was a recent Padovan invention—and here things would have gotten tricky. Unlike other prion disease sufferers, FFI victims have temperatures that gyrate wildly. The doctors would not have known what to make of these huge swings but they would have treated their friend as a fever victim anyway. (Part of clinical judgment consisted in knowing when to disregard results that didn't make sense.) They would ultimately have prescribed a soak in cold water—the servants desperately trying to hold his body so that he didn't slide under—and when that proved useless, they would have bled their friend to cool his humors, astonished by the jerking of his legs and arms as they tried to open the vein. Had they not been men of science, his condition would have looked to them more like possession than disease, but medicine had turned a corner in the last two hundred years and modern doctors such as they would never again talk of demons and auguries.

They would have convened again soon after, dressed in the black togas and soft velvet hats of their profession, probably in the card room in the doctor's house where over dinner and wine they would have debated what to do next. Purgatives? Emetics? Diuretics? None of the doctors would have been honest and said that they had no cure for their friend, because in reality none of them ever had a cure for anyone. In fact, no eighteenth-century doctors knew how to make a patient well; they had no more success than the mountebanks who lined the Piazza San Marco. They had all suffered humiliations similar to one Casanova recounts in his memoirs. The adventurer happened to be in a gondola with a Venetian patrician—a senator—when the man was felled by a stroke. Casanova helped the man into his palazzo and into bed, where he waited for the arrival of the senator's physician. A Dr. Ferro, eminent in the profession, arrived and placed a poultice or mercury salve on his patient's chest and left confident he would find him better in the morning. As he did—only to discover that in the night Casanova, seeing the senator near death from the cure (mercury is highly toxic) had stripped off the salve and washed his body in warm water. The patrician declared Casanova his new physician, and Casanova spread the story everywhere.

"Who is it that says there is a great difference between a good physician and a bad one; yet very little between a good one and none at all?" asked Arthur Young, the English agricultural journalist, in 1787, on a tour of the Continent. Still, faced with a sleepless, thrashing colleague, urged on by his terrified wife, the doctors would have taken action. In a case this grave, the best option was to prescribe the most powerful drug in their repertoire: *triaca,* or *teriaca,* or *theriaca ex Galena.* Or, in English, Venetian treacle.

Triaca was a typical Venetian story. Galen himself was said to have concocted the original version of the drug, and the recipe had then followed the Roman armies into Europe. With the collapse of the empire, its formula had survived in the monasteries: for the next fourteen hundred years, it remained the wonder drug of Europe. *Triaca* was reputed to cure fever and even the plague, and to counteract all poisons. The exact recipe varied depending on the ingredients available in the region and the druggist's tastes.

The Venetians had begun manufacturing *triaca* in the Middle Ages, taking advantage of their window on the east to fill it with ingredients to which other European countries didn't have access. By law, members of the *magistrato alla sanità,* the department of public health, had to be present when the apothecary ground and mixed these ingredients. The public was sometimes invited to attend too, the apothecary's shop with its impressive jars on burnished wood shelves an appealing locale for a show. Once the health department had certified the treacle as authentic, the druggist was allowed to hang the Venetian flag, the lion of Saint Mark the Evangelist, outside to alert the world that a new batch of treacle was on sale. The hocus-pocus of government certification turned treacle into a patented brand that Venice could ship to the rest of Europe at a good profit.

Treacle's most important ingredient was viper's flesh—"the base and foundation . . . without which you can absolutely not concoct it," as the great sixteenth-century Bolognese physician Aldrovandi wrote. The theory, enshrined in the work of Galen himself, was that it took a poison to counteract a poison. Since fever was a poison in the body, you needed an equally potent venom to stop it. The best (and most expensive) viper's flesh happened to come from the Euganean Hills near Padua, on Venetian territory.

The doctor's colleagues would have been able to negotiate a good price for the expensive drug because doctors licensed pharmacists in Venice. They would have carried the concoction back to their friend's house, where he now lay confined to his bed. They would have had to put the treacle paste directly on his tongue, bidding him to swallow it, or, if he was too weak to do so, they might have dissolved a small amount of the treacle in rose water to hide its bitter taste, and dripped it down his throat. Treacle is a diaphoretic, which means it makes the recipient sweat, the last thing a sufferer of fatal familial insomnia needs. And while the viper flesh likely had no effect, the opium with which treacle was laced certainly would have. The phrase "treacle sleep" appears in several European languages to mean a deep, dreamless sleep, but the opium in the doctor's brain would not have brought about that result. He would no longer have had the capacity in his brain for sleep, because prions had eaten it away. The opium would have eased his pain for a period, dulling the horror of what he experienced, but his eyes would have remained open.

After the treacle passed from his system, he would have been worse off than before, his servants having to hold his arms and legs down to keep him from twitching and jerking out of bed. Perhaps his wife would have given them permission to tie him down. Mutely, the doctor would have watched them do it.

All the same his colleagues would have declared themselves satisfied; the treacle had helped reduce their friend's phlegm: you had only to look at how sweaty he was. And from a professional point of view, who could fault them if the patient died, as he surely would soon? They had encountered a challenging case and devised a therapy, the best one available to them. And while medicine had progressed in the past century and would progress in the next, they were just men. Now it was the priests' turn.

In 1770, a man named Giuseppe was born in the Veneto. It is not clear exactly how he was related to the doctor; the family name was common by the eighteenth century, and citizens bearing it were "spread all over Venice," according to a contemporary document, but he may have been his nephew.

Giuseppe grew up in the doctor's country villa and may have inherited it at some point, though later he moved to a nearby town. He was a rural noble, a *siòr,* a man of property. He did not get to enjoy his privileged life for long, though. When he was in his late twenties, revolutionary France invaded Venice. Napoleon declared the Venetian Republic a meritocracy and suddenly everyone—patrician, doctor, lawyer, gondolier—became simply "cittadino." No sooner however had Venice accepted "Libertà Virtù Eguaglianza" than Napoleon traded the city to the Austrians for Belgium and Lombardy. Again the Venetians adjusted. "A Venetian law lasts but a week," one noble famously noted. Quickly the Venetians exchanged their red leggings, collars, and gloves (red was the color of the revolution) for black ones (the color of piety) and met the Austrians in the Piazza San Marco to celebrate mass for the Catholic emperor. Nine years later, Napoleon, now an emperor himself, was back; the Venetians put up his statue and a gilded "N" in Piazza San Marco, only to pull both down after his defeat at Waterloo in 1815. The victors of that battle, Austria, Britain, and Prussia, gave Venice back to Austria, which ruled it for another fifty years—except during a liberal insurrection in 1848—until it was absorbed by the new nation of Italy.

The days when a Venetian would crush his wife's pearls sooner than appear to bow before a foreign king were over. The great powers fought constantly on Venice's doorstep, carried off its grain, and blockaded its ports. Venice, bereft of its territories, suffered an economic collapse so severe it took a hundred years to recover.

The small towns that dotted the countryside of the Veneto, like the one Giuseppe lived in, were hit especially hard. The early Venetians had never cared about terra firma. Only in the fifteenth century did the Republic change its mind and, to protect itself, acquire possessions in territorial Italy. Not surprisingly, over time they learned to make quite a bit of money off their holdings. Not only did the towns serve the defense of the Republic, but they also functioned as an economic colony for the rich in their fantasy city across the lagoon. The peasants in the Veneto grew corn and ground it at mills along the rivers to ship to the capital, and raised silk worms whose cocoons the artisans in Venice could weave into the beautiful clothes of the Venetian rich. When those clothes were dirty, they were sent by boat back to the Veneto, where the locals washed and ironed them. A patrician could sit on the balcony of his country house in the Veneto and watch his clean laundry, his food, and his firewood go past on their way to his palazzo in the city.

When the fortunes of the aristocratic class fell, so did those of their support industries in the Veneto. The Veneto suffered further when, in an effort to satisfy their need for transportation across the countryside, the Venetians and then the Austrians began rerouting the shallow, winding network of rivers that carried water from the nearby mountains into the lagoon. This bit of hubris turned the Veneto into a swamp for much of the year. The swamp brought mosquitoes and the mosquitoes brought malaria; an 1849 Austrian military report stated that one quarter of the residents of Giuseppe's town had the debilitating, occasionally fatal disease. Malaria prevented peasants from farming, which in turn led to outbreaks of pellagra, a disease of malnutrition. One of the prime symptoms of pellagra was insanity and one of the prime symptoms of malaria is delirium and intermittent fever. As a result, the Veneto in the mid-nineteenth century was full of people who had symptoms that resembled fatal familial insomnia.

Of Giuseppe's eight children, five died before reaching their first birthday. So much infant death was in line with the norms of country life, even among the wealthy, and Giuseppe would have accepted it. He would, however, have been surprised when, in about 1827, his teenaged son Costante became ill. At first the boy's fever would have come and gone, but within a few months he would have begun hallucinating and maybe claiming he was possessed. The local witch, an old spinster who lived on the edge of town, would have been brought in. Her solution would have been to shine light in every corner of Costante's sleeping quarters, in order to repel the *massarió,* the malicious elf who liked to surprise sleepers in the middle of the night by sitting on their chests, making them gasp for air. Or she might have taken Costante into the countryside and swung him three times under a chestnut tree, a cure-all.

When Costante didn't get better, Giuseppe would have tried a local priest—there were priests in the Veneto reputed to be able to return the mad to their senses. At the altar of the town church, beneath swirling frescoes of the baptism of Christ executed by one of Tiepolo's sons, the priest would have sprinkled holy water on Costante and had him touch the cross. When that didn't work, he would have locked the boy in the church with him and performed an exorcism. Exorcism was back-breaking labor, but no matter how much the priest sweated to remove this devil, Costante would have sweated more.

The boy died in 1828. The parish priest recorded his cause of death as pellagra, although the assertion makes no sense—pellagra was a disease of the poor, and Giuseppe's family was rich. But Giuseppe would not have had long to think about the priest's error. Soon, he fell sick too. He might not have associated his disease with his son's, though, because FFI manifests itself differently depending on the age of the victim: in younger sufferers it causes mental disorders, while in older ones its primary symptom is insomnia. Giuseppe's disease would have resembled those of his forebear, the Venetian doctor—the sweating, the fevers, most of all, the sleeplessness.

"*Tempo, siori, dotori i fa chelo che i voli lori*"—"Time, gentlemen, and doctors do what they want" went a local saying. Still, in his mid-fifties, a *capofamiglia*, a *siòr* himself, Giuseppe would have called on *il medico*. He would not have found relief there, though. The doctor would have diagnosed malaria. He might have prescribed quinine— Giuseppe could have afforded the very expensive drug—but it would not have helped. In the fifty years since the Venetian doctor's death, considerable new medical knowledge had come to the fore: physicians now knew that people breathed oxygen and that nerves carried both sensory and motor impulses for instance. But FFI remained vastly beyond the medical competency of the time. Giuseppe died shortly after Costante, his disease also a mystery.

In retrospect, with our knowledge of how the mutation in Giuseppe's genes would spread and what misery it would bring, it might have been better if instead of having killed five of his children in infancy, disease had taken all eight, because with Angelo and Vincenzo, his two children who survived to adulthood, the mutation began to spread. Both men are obligate carriers—that is, the pattern of those who have the FFI mutation today indicates that both brothers must have had it. Angelo, who was born in 1813, died of FFI, probably sometime in the 1870s, and Vincenzo, born in 1822, died of cancer of the lip before the disease could strike, in 1880.

Angelo had one child, of whom we know nothing. About Vincenzo we know more, because his branch of the family, the one Lisi descends from, made a family tree. Vincenzo was a farmer—the parish books list him as *contadino,* or peasant, though he likely owned his own land, having inherited it from Giuseppe. His wife, Marianna, known for her full mane of red hair, survived him, and in her widowhood, she drove around in a sporty one-horse carriage called a calèche, visiting her many children. It was a lucky mother who saw six of her eight children to adulthood as she had, and when she died in 1893, in the back room of her villa with its view of the sun setting behind the Dolomites, she had reason to believe that she had lived a blessed life.

But of her and Vincenzo's six descendants, four probably died from FFI: Angelo in his mid-thirties in 1901, Pierina in her early forties in 1906, Giovanni in his mid-forties in 1913, and Antonio in his mid-fifties in 1926. For each, a different cause of death is named in the parish book—from dementia to pellagra. Also, at around this time a plague engulfed Europe: encephalitis lethargica, or Von Economo's disease. Its main symptom was either insomnia or endless sleepiness. At autopsy, encephalitis lethargica victims evinced swelling of the brain, but autopsy was still something only the poorest of the poor endured. So, many family members who died of FFI in this period were lumped in with the millions who, by chance, briefly joined them on their sleepless odyssey.

In later years, when family members came to understand what had happened to them, they would blame Marianna for the disease—"the accursed redhead," Lisi's mother would call her. Perhaps she was blamed because her family was not from the Veneto. Or it may have been because she had red hair, and family members believed that those who had red hair were more likely to come down with the malady. But she was not the carrier: her husband, Vincenzo, was.

Starting with their children, FFI followed an unfortunate pattern. Those branches that carried the mutation grew poorer, because they kept losing able-bodied adults. In response, like most poor families, they tended to have extra children to help with their labor, and as a hedge against high infant mortality rates. Because large families tend to suffer more from genetic diseases, those branches with the mutation fell further. Meanwhile, the branches that had escaped the mutation hurried to put distance between themselves and their sick cousins. Disease was a matter of particularly intense shame in the Veneto, and in the malarial swamp that was the region in this period, families necessarily judged men and women for their fitness. Did the young woman have wide hips helpful in giving birth? Did the young man appear too sickly to bring in the harvest? Did tuberculosis run in his family? There was so much worry about being branded as diseased that the sick would start on the road out of town and then circle back around so their neighbors didn't see them visiting the town doctor.

The high death rate in the Venetan countryside finally began to subside at the beginning of the twentieth century, thanks to land reclamation projects and emigration (four million Venetans left for the Americas). But as things got better around them, the plight of Vincenzo's descendants grew starker. Their neighbors, aware that many members of the family had died strange deaths before reaching sixty, began to think twice about marrying into the family. Some of Vincenzo's progeny died bachelors or spinsters in the Veneto; others left for America, Switzerland, France—places where they would not be known and could start again. Those who stayed put on a brave face and never spoke about the family problem to outsiders. Even among themselves, they referred to the disease obliquely. It was a disease of exhaustion or stress, brought on by sorrow or loss. It was never characterized as something over which they had no control, something that lay dormant in their bodies waiting to strike them down and then their descendants. They were alone now in their misery, sufferers of a unique disease—or so they believed.

CHAPTER 2

MERINO MANIA ENGLAND, *1772*

Machines for converting herbage . . . into money.

—ROBERT BAKEWELL, on sheep

Around the same time the Venetian doctor was dying, another prion disease was breaking out across Europe. The continent's prize flocks of sheep were falling victim to a strange new syndrome. The disease came to be called scrapie, after its most pronounced symptom. Ordinarily, sheep are docile, uninterested, and uninteresting creatures—if shepherds didn't have pipes (or, in modern times, radios), they would fall asleep tending them. But when a sheep gets scrapie, its behavior changes. It becomes aggressive and high-strung, charging or fleeing at the sight of a sheepdog or the sound of a whistle. And tickling a scrapie-infected animal under the chin will cause it to smack its lips noisily—something sheep don't ordinarily do. The oddest thing about a scrapie-infected sheep is that it seems to go crazy trying to scratch an unrelenting, imaginary itch. Feeling this itch most acutely on its back and the top of its tail, the sheep will scrape these parts bloody against posts, walls, rocks—against anything it can find—looking for relief. In reality the itchiness is caused by alterations in the sheep's brain brought on by prions, and no amount of scratching at the skin can soothe it. But by the time a scrapie-afflicted sheep dies—the disease is always fatal— its back and rump are raw and scabbed over and its fleece is in tatters.

Scrapie remains a problem today almost everywhere in the world. *La tremblante, le vertigo, der Traberkrankheit* (the trotting disease)— a word for it exists in nearly every European language and many others besides. There is evidence that scrapie always existed in the countryside, but it was never a serious agricultural problem until a new generation of men and their ideas—in particular, the idea to make sheep more profitable through intensive breeding—put it on the map.

By the eighteenth century, what nature had placed on the earth had begun to seem inadequate to Europeans. Surely, there were ways to improve what they saw. Could farm animals be bigger? Could they be made to eat less? Could they be bred in a way that increased the meat on their frames and decreased the bone? Lending urgency to such thinking was the remarkable growth of the continent's population— England alone had almost three times as many people in 1850 as in 1750; the country's farms had to feed a lot more mouths. Intelligent minds of the sort that congregated in London coffeehouses disagreed over whether this was possible. They turned to Adam Smith's *Wealth of Nations,* published in 1776, for an answer. Smith's theory that the invisible hand of the market helped keep society's supply and demand in balance worked perfectly for manufactured goods. But in the world of agriculture, as many pointed out, the market didn't play quite the same role. Britain, an island nation, was not growing, and the amount of food each English acre produced could not be increased indefinitely. A rising population would create more demand for food, as Smith predicted, but the consequent price increase would not (because it could not) lead to vastly increased production. The result would be famine.

This was the opinion of the age's reigning pessimist, Thomas Malthus. A professor at Cambridge, Malthus came from a rich London family and had no great compassion for the poor. ("Unless Mr. Malthus can contrive to starve someone," commented the critic William Hazlitt, "he thinks he does nothing.") But he had a point, one even Adam Smith could appreciate: famine was a classic if brutal manifestation of the hidden hand.

Overall though, the temper of the times was optimistic. "The age we live in is a busy age," wrote the political philosopher Jeremy Bentham, "in which knowledge is rapidly advancing towards perfection. In the natural world, in particular, every thing teems with discovery and with improvement." There was a sizable school of noblemen and intellectuals who, thanks to the wealth the industrial revolution was generating for them, believed they could fulfill Bentham's aspirations in the field. Specifically, they thought it might be possible to make land already under cultivation more productive.

Agricultural productivity became a great cause of the second half of the eighteenth century, not just in England but across Europe. It linked all the themes of the Enlightenment—the power of reason and the idea that man was born good; the acknowledgment that he was also naturally greedy, and the possibility that that greed might be a virtue. What was more, providing adequate food—especially meat—to the growing populations of one's native land was a patriotic act. One had only to look at the bread riots and the political unrest in France to understand the connection between political stability and food supply.

The spirit of the age found its exemplar in Robert Bakewell, a talented livestock breeder with a drive to make money. Bakewell farmed outside the town of Dishley, in Leicester, about a hundred miles north of London. Like most English farmers, he did not own his fields; a rich Londoner did. Bakewell was, in the parlance of the day, a common farmer, but class meant little to him. What mattered was money and, critically for the story of sheep and their diseases, he had a remarkable ability to see that there was more money to be made in what walked on the land than in what grew from it. England's cities were exploding with a new working class, which had an enormous appetite for mutton that it could not afford.

The worker generally had to content himself with scraps of meat in his soup—he rarely got a joint. This, Bakewell realized, was because English farm animals were skinny, ill-formed, and heavy-boned. They carried their meat in the wrong places, and required an enormous amount of pasture to give back small returns. They were, in short, "unthrifty"—Bakewell's strongest condemnation.

He believed he could change this equation. The perfect sheep, he thought, would have a tiny head, a small neck, skinny legs, and an enormous breast and rump (somewhat like the modern industrial farm turkey). Animals were not God's creation but man's—they were bred to be slaughtered, sold, and eaten. This was Bakewell's great insight. It was also a key source for the spread of scrapie.

Bakewell knew that to improve farm animals, you had to start with animals that already had a tendency to do what you wanted them to do—to grow fat quickly. Of course, if remaking nature had been easy to do, someone would have done it before. But breeding was difficult. Even Darwin, who would later use the success Bakewell and his followers had with artificial selection to posit natural selection—evolution— recognized this fact: "Not one man in a thousand has accuracy of eye and judgement sufficient to become an eminent breeder," he noted in *The Origin of Species.* Robert Bakewell was that man.

Most remarkable about his breeding technique was how he made it up as he went along. Neither he nor anyone else in his day really understood the mechanism of inheritance. But Bakewell knew what he saw with his own eyes—that rams and ewes passed on their body types to their offspring and that, often, they passed on traits that occurred together; for instance, sheep with small bones also tended to put on weight quickly. But most of all, Bakewell succeeded at his project because he had a genius for selecting which sheep to breed. By the 1740s, his sheep were already getting bigger and meatier. When he had a winning sheep—out of a generation of rams, he only allowed a handful to go to stud; he had no tolerance for losers—he bred it with its own offspring, again and again, until the genetic contribution of one parent in its offspring might reach 95 percent. The process was called breeding in-and-in. It was nothing that had been in wide practice before, because it contravened the wisdom of farmers, which was that inbreeding brought out hereditary defects in animals. Breeding in-and-in also touched the same nerve that cloning does today: for some it violated a sense of the natural order. Bakewell and his followers, Richard Parkinson, an agricultural writer, complained, were "setting themselves in opposition to their Creator by endeavouring to destroy his works."

Bakewell did not care, and his results began to amaze his neighbors. He remade the scraggly indigenous breed of the Leicester into a phenomenon. Renamed the Dishley Leicester, it was barrel-chested, with spindly legs and a tiny head, looking like a water tank on four legs. He announced that he had "substitute[d] profitable flesh for useless bone." Even Malthus was impressed.

With his farm on the main road to London, Bakewell's achievements were just poised for discovery by a larger audience. A turning point came in 1771 when Arthur Young, the most celebrated agricultural writer of his age, paid him a visit. Young had the ear of the king, and his books were best-sellers. What followed was a mutual admiration society heavily colored by self-interest. Young called Bakewell "the Prince of Breeders." Bakewell named his favorite ram after Young.

Drawn by Young's publicity, the famous now came to call on Bakewell. In 1788 the king himself, who liked to style himself "Farmer George," warmly welcomed the breeder to St. James' Palace. Young reported that they spoke for more than an hour. With the mark of His Majesty's approval, Bakewell now became even better known—and richer. One year he made £1,200 (£150,000 in contemporary money) from the stud fees paid him for a single ram.

Bakewell tried to form combines with those who had bred using his Dishley Leicesters to keep prices high, but he couldn't control the progress he had wrought. He had become a movement, a mind-set, a bellwether; thousands followed him. Anyone with a claim to being a modern breeder began breeding his sheep in-and-in, whether he began with Bakewell's sheep or other stock. To do otherwise was to defy the national goal of self-sufficiency, and lose money, too. In 1710 the average sheep weighed twenty-eight pounds at Smithfield market in London, the average lamb eighteen pounds. By 1795, the year of Bakewell's death, the average weight for a sheep was eighty pounds and for a lamb fifty. The descendants of Bakewell's Dishley Leicesters changed the breeds of England and, ultimately, those of Europe and the Americas down to the present day; modern sheep look a lot like Bakewell's sheep and less like their seventeenth-century forebears.

Bakewell and his followers improved the lives of the fast-growing working class too. For the first time, meat was available year-round in the markets of the big cities, and the poor no longer got only scraps. Why was there no revolution in Britain to echo the one in France? In part because of Bakewell and those who learned from him. What Bakewell called "the cause" helped maintain Britain's peace.

Even so, the gentry of England were not thrilled with Bakewell's success. They had an intuition that what he was doing was not ultimately in their interest. They began to attack him, insisting he'd ruined the taste of the meat. An anonymous critic wrote that Bakewell's mutton was "only fit to glide down the throat of a Newcastle coalheaver." One of Bakewell's key opponents was Sir Joseph Banks, the president of the Royal Society. Banks was an important man, effectively the king's chief science advisor. Himself a sheep owner, Banks did not like Bakewell, rarely missing an opportunity to denigrate him. Still, the two had something in common; like Bakewell, Banks had a sheep project in the works, although Banks's involved wool. Many of the mills popping up along English streams and rivers knit textiles. In some regions, a quarter of the population did work connected to the mills, making cloth for trousers, blankets, and jackets. The mills were ravenous for a good fiber count, which could only come from superior sheep.

But in this regard, Britain was far behind its primary competitor, Spain. Spanish wool was so good that English manufacturers paid more than a million pounds a year to import it. And increased demand was causing increased prices.

With eighteen million sheep in England, the situation was in some ways quite shameful. Worse yet, England was a sworn political enemy of Spain. "To depend upon a Country naturally unkindly to you for the Raw material of the finest branch of your Principal manufacture & to be in hourly danger of the privilege of Obtaining it being resumd is a humiliating consideration to a great nation," Banks pointed out in a note to the king in 1788.

Banks knew that the excellence of the sheep of Spain was not an accident. For centuries, the Spanish had bred their best sheep, called merinos, with exquisite judgment. Their flocks, some five million strong, were under the care of the Mesta, a private body chartered by the king and given the extraordinary right to graze their sheep practically anywhere they wanted. Each winter the Mesta shepherds drove the merinos from the mountains of Castile to the hot plains of Estremadura along twelve thousand miles of special roads, then drove them back the following fall. Boys inherited the job of shepherd from their fathers, and they grew up eyeing sheep flesh, learning to evaluate which traits should be encouraged and which bred out.

The result of five centuries of careful breeding was a wondrous-looking creature: narrow with a full chest and wild topknots of fur (what a contemporary English observer called "a peculiar coarse and unsightly growth of hair on the forehead and cheeks"), wrinkles on the neck ("a singular looseness of the skin"), and so much grease on their fleeces they looked as if they'd been dipped in batter. But once a merino was sheared and the wool cleaned, it was clear how special it was. Its wool was finer, suppler, springier, simply the best in the world. Once knit, its elegant sheen was unmistakable.

It had long been obvious not just to the British but to the rest of Europe that having some merinos to breed with would improve the wool of their own flocks. The problem though was that Spain would not export them—in fact, Mesta members were subject to arrest if they crossed a border with their sheep. This would have seemed the end of that, but Banks was an enterprising man and the king was insistent.

So Banks sought ways around the embargo. He used British merchants, Spanish "contrabandays," and his friendship with a French agronomist to wheedle, bribe, and trade for a few dozen merino sheep. Once in England, the sheep did not thrive. Banks thought the problem might be the climate or maybe the king's shepherds, who did not seem interested in the extra work necessary to care for the merinos. Again and again Banks and the king went to see the sheep, pastured at Kew Palace and Windsor, only to be informed of another death. Almost 25 percent of the merinos died in 1795 and 1796; 28 percent of those left died a year later. The toll among the rams, valuable for their ability to breed widely, was more than a third. Those that survived were in a poor state.

And yet the merinos found takers. Banks sold them carefully to landowners who had enough sheep to get the breed going. Roughly thirty-five aristocrats received a merino directly in the first years of the merino project. Royal employees ferried them—they were too fragile to walk—from the king's pastures to their new homes. All too often, though, Banks dispatched a sheep as a gift from His Majesty, and Lord So-and-So wrote back politely to say that the animal had arrived dead at his door.

Even with those that got there alive, there was no time to waste.

Few merinos were lasting more than three years. Although the elite still disdained Bakewell, they had taken note of his innovation: if you wanted to change the make-up of a flock quickly, you had to breed in-and-in. Banks had deliberately spread the king's merinos across much of England; now their recipients set about making sure their thick top-knots and batter-dipped wool did not disappear. Landowners bred them with their local breeds and then bred them again with their own offspring and their offspring's offspring. A merino ram might be both great-great-great-grandfather and father to its own descendant. The merino crosses, as the descendants were called (though many were nearly pure merinos, due to the inbreeding), were in turn shipped out to other landowners to spread their desirable traits.

In 1802, Arthur Young could write that there were merinos "in almost every district of Great Britain." And the aristocrats were breeding the hell out of them. Who could blame them? They had been waiting more than five centuries for the chance. They might be forgiven for not considering the consequences.

Thomas Comber, a clergyman in Huntingdonshire, was the first to record the new problem. The year was 1772. Banks had not yet assembled his flock, but Bakewell and his descendants had been breeding in-and-in for some thirty years by then.

Though a man of the church, Comber was deeply interested in farming. He was in the habit of wandering the countryside on "daily Excursions," ostensibly for his health, but really to satisfy this curiosity. He had read and absorbed Arthur Young's books—even had a mostly one-sided correspondence with him—and Young was often on his mind on these walks, Comber's conservative nature making him something of a rebutter to the celebrated agricultural writer with his passion for progress. The clergyman found the new preference for horses over oxen ill conceived, and he disapproved of the modern enthusiasm for young mutton. "No person who has taste," he wrote, "can doubt that the mutton of a four shear sheep is preferable to that of a three shear sheep (*caet par.*)."

One day about a year after he had arrived in Huntingdonshire, Comber happened upon a parishioner who told him something disturbing about his sheep. Thomas Beal lived in Morborne, the smaller of Comber's two parishes, where he was the principal farmer. He was rich and forward-looking enough to have bought a stud bull from Robert Bakewell for twelve guineas.

Beal mentioned that some of his sheep were falling sick, and in a way he had not seen before. They seemed to suffer a terrible itch. They were always rubbing their backsides and the tops of their head behind the ears against fence stakes, barn walls, stable posts, even their own hooves. But the itch seemed incurable, and, in the disease's later stages, the animals teetered, tumbled, stumbled, and ultimately fell down dead. Deaths from the disease had cost Beal several hundred pounds.

Sheep and disease were no strangers to each other. Braxy, thwarter-ill, the black lights, liver-fluke, and rot were just a few of their afflictions. For every disease in the farmyard, there was a supposed cure too—turpentine, tobacco, tincture of mercury, or dew-cup mixed with merry leaf. Yet the disease afflicting Beal's sheep stood out. For one thing, it was quickly lethal. Between the first sign of illness and death there passed only a couple of months. For another, the sickness seemed to be spreading: according to Beal, the disease had become general in the county in the past forty years. Farmers called it rickets, after the disease that left children's legs weakened. Rickets in humans had been diagnosed in Europe only about a hundred years before, so it seemed reasonable to ask whether the relatively new disease was also appearing in sheep. But farmers weren't doctors, and no one had really taken up the question.

Comber was intrigued. He had never heard of this problem. He knew a new disease of sheep was not just a curiosity—it had the potential to be economically devastating, if it was spreading as quickly as Beal suggested. Comber found out more. He had asked Beal how he knew whether sheep had the disease. Beal had said that at first their sexual appetites ran wild. They also got a distant look in their eyes and refused to stand with the flock, holding their heads oddly, in what James Hogg, a veterinary writer, described as "a fixed and convulsed position." As the disease progressed, the sheep were sometimes so tired they would stand still with their heads resting on the ground. Farmers had tried many of their home cures on this disease, but none had worked. Usually the sheep died at night, in the cold or in a rain.

Comber laboriously wrote down these points in his notebook. Then he sat down and addressed a letter to Dr. Alexander Hunter, a physician and acquaintance of his from his old parish in York. Hunter, the editor of the agricultural journal there and a member of Banks's Royal Society, had once honored Comber with a copy of his *Georgical Essays*. Now Comber put on his best medical voice, and dividing into three parts his observations on a new "Distemper among Sheep, very dreadful to every Lover of Agriculture," described the symptoms and asked for help: "That if the philosophy, Sir, of you and your learned brethren can assist us, a cure may be found; and if not, that the farmer may be taught by good authority to give up vain hopes of a cure, and to quit the whole breed as soon as possible, and not lose time and money by vain attempts after one."

The process of scientific discovery, then as now, was full of politics. Hunter appears to have ignored Comber's letter. But Comber was not easily discouraged. He had come from a family of some reputation— his grandfather, a Cambridge vice-chancellor, had defied Cromwell— and he had the reputation to get the word out. The potential economic impact of what he was hearing was too important to keep from the general public. He got a London printer and bookseller who had been one of Young's publishers to print his "rickets" letter and staked his claim to a new disease.

Soon Comber's "dreadful malady" was all over England; by the early 1800s, it had reached Scotland, where by mid-century farmers called it "scrapie." Awareness of agricultural disease was local—as local as food or language—and elsewhere scrapie went under an assortment of names: rubbers and euky pine, the frenzies, the giddies, scratchie, shrewcroft (meaning "evil place"), turnsick, the dizzies, the shaking, and the "cuddy-trot" ("cuddies" were ponies). The most frequent term was "goggles," either from Gloucestershire dialect for "giddies" or from observation of the effect the disease has on an afflicted sheep's eyes. "I dare say," Comber had written Hunter, "if his Eye-balls were examined, they would appear inflamed."

Britain did not have a central scientific or health authority to spread the word of the new outbreak; Banks, as head of the Royal Society, came closest to fulfilling that role, but he would not talk about goggles. No doubt he knew what the rumor of infection could do to his flock's commercial prospects, and to the king's admiration of him. As for Young, whose own flock was decimated by scrapie, he also said little. "*Quere* this?" he wrote in the *Annals of Agriculture* of 1793, "for it is very curious." Consequently we can only guess at the extent of the English scrapie outbreak, though a manuscript prepared a century later by an Oxford professor of veterinary medicine, H. B. Parry, estimated that 5 percent to 10 percent of Britain's sheep were affected. The number may have been much higher.

Estimating the size of the outbreak is particularly hard because shepherds—as they do today—took great pains to hide its presence. Herding was a solitary profession, graziers the bane of the tax man: no accounting books, little in the way of barns and equipment, a constantly changing head count. Shepherds, alone and bored in the fields, were excellent detectives. A shepherd would notice "shrugginess"— the telltale stiff posture and inattentiveness characteristic of scrapie's onset—long before a buyer would, and could easily kill that sheep or claim it had wandered off. As Comber pointed out, breeders who dumped sick sheep at market courted "Infamy and a prosecution at Law," but that did not stop them. A prize sheep might be worth £1,500, or $185,000—$270,000 in modern terms. Even an ordinary breeding ram could command a couple of hundred pounds at auction. Once such an animal showed signs of scrapie, he was just mutton.

As soon as scrapie broke out in Comber's district and the surrounding areas, aristocrats pointed a finger at Bakewell and his breeding practices. A landowner in Somersetshire wrote to Banks in 1800 to accuse Bakewell and his cronies of "bad taste & unnatural pride in crossing for large size." He claimed he could trace scrapie to a core stock of sheep that Bakewell had supposedly brought over from Holland. It is unlikely that he actually had the goods. For one thing, Bakewell covered his tracks well: he was very secretive during his life, and his records disappeared with his death. (Banks once sent a friend to poke around about Bakewell's breeding techniques, only to find the man's contact, a shepherd, had fallen down a well.) What's more, Bakewell was a perceptive businessman. At the first sign of disease, one can be sure he would have destroyed the afflicted sheep. "The only way to have capital stock is to keep the price high," he liked to say. Rumors of disease in his flock would not advance that cause. And Bakewell may not even have known that scrapie was spreading from his flocks: he shipped his rams out to breed long before the disease would have manifested itself. No matter, breeding in-and-in was a recipe for disaster, and Bakewell knew it.

Landowners hoped Banks's Spanish merinos would help to eradicate scrapie in their flocks by bringing in new blood, but in fact Banks's project appears to have worsened the problem, because some of his merinos had scrapie as well. His shepherds' logs are dotted with references to "goggles" and the "mad staggers." In 1798, at the annual shearing, Banks noted a "goggly" sheep and "ordered him to be killd." A ewe with goggles two years later was killed "as she was so weak that when down she could not rise." Banks's problems would not have surprised the Spanish. As one German agricultural writer noted, the "trotting disease in sheep" was "well known in Spain. But they have discovered no remedy for it as yet. Be it a sheep or a ram that begins to be affected with it, the Spaniards kill it immediately."

Banks and the king at one point suspected that the merino health problems might not have been an accident—their Spanish contacts had sent diseased sheep in order to foil the English in their efforts to produce better wool. That explanation would be more credible if nations friendlier to Spain had had a better experience with the Spanish merino. In fact they didn't. Over time the Spanish relaxed their prohibition on exporting merinos—politically weakened, the nation needed allies. The French king was among the beneficiaries and received several shipments, all diseased. And in Prussia, another beneficiary of the Spanish merino shipments via its possession of Silesia, the disease became enough of a problem that a sixty-eight-page manual was printed in Breslau detailing the outbreak.

By the 1820s, scrapie threatened to destroy the continent's mutton and wool businesses. What's more, it challenged the generally positive trend that seemed to be making life more pleasant—the increasing harvests and fatter sheep that made even the pessimistic Malthus rethink the certainty of human starvation in the second edition of his *Essay on Population.*

The Enlightenment impulse was not to be contained; from the beginning, men thought they could understand the disease. Theories proliferated about its causes and cures. In what is probably the first mention of scrapie in English, Thomas Fuller, an Anglican bishop writing in 1642, suggested mixing goats in with afflicted sheep to stop the disease. Edward Lisle, an English aristocrat who at the end of the seventeenth century retreated to Hampshire and, much like Thomas Comber, filled his time chatting with farmers, recommended milk cows for the same purpose. The French thought you could cure scrapie with one gram of verlaine and twenty grams of camphor, while Banks and Young trusted in arsenic and mercury, the Spanish in sulfur smoke, pepper, and pork fat, and the Germans in stinking hellebore, an evergreen.

The problem was not that these theories of scrapie and its cure were wrong. It was that the basic scientific knowledge necessary to judge them hadn't yet cohered. Toward the end of the eighteenth century, universities created their first chairs in veterinary medicine, a move that gave the field a considerable boost—and by the mid-nineteenth century, in an era when an animal might be worth more than the farmer who tended it, veterinary techniques came close to surpassing those of human medicine. But veterinary medicine also shared with human medicine a lack of the settled ideas that form the core of any medical or scientific effort. Were infections living things? Was every infection malevolent? When a living thing got sick, what exactly caused its death? Was it the invading force, the damage that force did to the body, or the shock it caused the animal? Science had not yet separated itself from natural philosophy. "Disease is that deviation from health, which, in a greater or lesser degree, disorders the frame and spirits, yielding either to some critical effort of Nature or of Art, or, by its unremitting resistance, destroying the fabric by producing death," wrote Charles Vial de Sainbel, one of the first veterinarians, in 1797.

Formulations like this one were elegant dead ends. They did not clarify what made a living thing susceptible to disease, or why if two people (or two flocks) were exposed to the same disease, only one might get sick. One medieval scholar had posed a question that still didn't have much of an answer: if you can catch a disease, why can't you catch a cure? Contagion was a vague concept. It was something—a force or a body—that transferred disease or caused its transfer into a living entity. That force or body might itself be living or dead, or perhaps a bit of both, like fetid swamp air (the supposed cause of malaria). Rarely were these gropings sufficient to solve the mystery of what caused a given disease, and when it came to scrapie, this confusion proved overwhelming. (Even twenty-first-century researchers have had only limited success in unraveling its unusual mixture of genetic and infectious causes.)

Some blamed scrapie on malarial air, while others blamed it on the wind or overheated sheep pens. Some thought too much food brought on the symptoms; others, too little—or an abrupt change in pasturage. For yet others, direct sunlight was responsible for the disease. In 1772, Thomas Beal proposed that the cause of scrapie was maggots. Beal had been convinced that the insect entered through the nose, and once in the head, went on to embed itself in the brain. While it was true, others pointed out, that scrapie sheep had maggots in their brains, so did non-scrapie sheep.

Still, the idea that insects caused scrapie was appealing. Sheep in general were infested animals, and the maggot theory gave scrapie a visible cause—or, at least, a nearly visible one. At the same time as Beal was finding maggots in his scrapie-infested sheep, a French professor of rural economy named Hénon successfully removed a worm from a sheep with scrapie. Soon after, the professor noted, the sheep "regained his gaiety and his appetite."

Both Young and Banks agreed that an insect was responsible, probably after reading the work of A.K.S. Von Richthofen, a Silesian baron and agricultural expert. Von Richthofen, a forebear of the Red Baron of World War I, saw scrapie as a double-barreled threat—first to the merino wool industry, which Silesia had jump-started with the import of some sheep from Spain, and second, to the food supply, since, as he pointed out, wealthier nations like his own consumed a lot of mutton while poor ones, like France, ate beef. Von Richthofen believed he'd found a mite, which he called the trotting-mite, that irritated the sheep's skin, producing the loss of fleece, the nervousness, "and in short order the other lethal aspects of the disease." The mite took twelve days from infection to outbreak and could be passed in nasal mucus—"green and white slime"—or during sexual intercourse, emerging intact in the skin of the offspring.

Von Richthofen's solution accounted admirably for how the disease could have two methods of spreading: infectious and inherited. The mite crossed from animal to animal just as the scabies mite did in sheep and lice did in humans. This was infection. At the same time, the mite could be transmitted to the ewe and from there to her offspring through copulation. Thus the disease traveled in families.

What the baron did not understand was the distinction between inherited disease and sexually transmitted disease. In this, he was not alone: no one knew how hereditary information was transferred from generation to generation (Darwin, for instance, thought the information was in the blood). Because of this confusion, genetic diseases were often ascribed to sexual causes. Von Richthofen's collaborator, M. Augustin, working in Potsdam, believed that scrapie was the result of excessive mating or mating too quickly and was passed on to offspring conceived in excessive heat. He thought it significant that the tail and the base of the spine, where the infection first manifested itself, were so close to the genitals.

For the French, excess copulation was not the explanation. In fact, just the opposite. They had noted that the most virile rams—literally, the "horniest"—tended to get the disease in disproportionate numbers. The reason was clearly sexual frustration, the pent-up semen causing scrapie in their offspring. The cure was to give the rams a chance to work off their excessive energies with some docile milk sheep before being led in to mate for real.

This proposition was supported by the observation that scrapie-afflicted sheep first became excessively lusty (human sufferers of prion diseases also sometimes initially experience increased sex drive, a result of the destruction of the system by which the body keeps its basic functions in balance). Yet over time it became clear that the sexual frustration link wasn't quite there. "We cannot figure out how violent ardor, incompletely satisfied, can cause a spinal neuralgic infection," wrote J. Girard, the much respected director of the newly founded Royal Veterinary School at Alfort.

While the theorists continued to speculate, the anatomists went at the corpses of sheep, confident they would find the answer to this mysterious disease with their more empiric techniques. They were to be disappointed. Some veterinarians thought they saw "tumours of a size varying from that of a green bean to that of a nut, or even to that of a hen's egg," others a lesion in the genital-urinary tract, and still others a clear pattern of cysts in the ovaries.

Perhaps no one was prouder of his profession than the French veterinarian Roche-Lubin. Roche-Lubin practiced in the mid-nineteenth century in Aveyron, an underdeveloped region in the foothills of the French Pyrenees, where he used the gospel of science to overcome "the ignorant simplicity or superstitious credulity of our luckless farmers." Scrapie was a favorite study of Roche-Lubin. To determine its cause, he slaughtered a group of sheep in different stages of the disease and opened them up right on the farm, only to find that their organs seemed completely normal. His precise anatomical investigations had netted him nothing—"*ni ulcères, ni vésicules, ni pustules, ni rougeurs, ni rien,*" as a colleague put it. After the disappointment of the autopsies, he fell back on a theory of scrapie as primitive as any he had spent his lifetime decrying. The "true causes" of scrapie, he wrote in 1848, were "excessive copulation, brutal combat among sheep, sustained ingestion of spicy foods, excessive leaping, violent exertions in general, fleeing pursuing dogs, claps of thunder, and forced isolation in the days immediately after shearing."

Roche-Lubin was so confident he had cracked the mystery that he tried to bring on the disease himself in sheep and then cure it. He gave a concoction of oats, bran, salt, pepper, viper-powder herb, blood-dragon herb, and ginger to a flock of forty dairy ewes. Much to his satisfaction, eight days later, nineteen of the sheep had come down with scrapie. Then Roche-Lubin gave them a dose of an anti-spasmodic drug. At first the drug seemed to work beautifully, but then the sheep sickened and died. J. Girard was not surprised by such results. "*Nous avons énoncé notre opinion sur son incurabilité,*" he wrote from Alfort. Or, as Arthur Young put it with admirable taciturnity, "the *rubbers,* a sort of itch; they rub themselves to death; no cure."

What ended the great scrapie epizootic of the early 1800s was the same force that had started it, the market. Joseph Banks was a man of many projects and through one of them he helped found the English colony of Australia. And when Australia, with its millions of acres of grassland and its lower farming costs, got into the sheep business in the mid-nineteenth century, the European sheep industry collapsed. Breeding sheep in-and-in no longer had an economic payoff, and with the pressure of artificial breeding off, breeds resistant to scrapie began to dominate flocks again. Scrapie did not disappear, but it became a low-level problem, "an obscure disease of sheep" as the title of an English research paper put it in 1913.

In the meantime, humankind finally agreed on a theory of contagion. In the 1860s and 1870s, Louis Pasteur and Robert Koch showed that living germs were the cause of infection, vanquishing the competing ideas that disease was caused by an imbalance of humors or contained in putrid air. Veterinarians reasonably assumed that scrapie could be understood within this new paradigm if anyone ever had the resources and took the time to try.

CHAPTER 3

PIETRO THE VENETO, *1943*

The doctor says it's useless, but I don't believe it because Papa
seems so healthy otherwise. What is this horrible disease?

—LETTER FROM ONE OF
PIETRO'S DAUGHTERS

The beginning of the twentieth century was a hopeful time in the Veneto. Italy was finally catching up to its European neighbors. Industrial growth in the cities and emigration had begun to draw peasants off the land, in turn raising the wages of farm laborers. The government ran huge hydraulic pumps that drained the swamps, sprayed vast quantities of pesticides, and distributed millions of doses of quinine, finally ending malaria's centuries-long dominance.

These advances passed by the descendants of the Italian doctor. While most Venetans heard a melody of progress, the doctor's family still heard the drumbeat of death. Vincenzo and Marianna's oldest son,

Giovanni, had twelve children of his own, at least eight of whom lived to adulthood. Of these eight, six probably died of fatal familial insomnia. The second of those was Pietro, born in 1894.

Pietro was handsome, with light-colored eyes, a strong jaw, and Marianna's bright red hair. He was born poor but learned to read and write in school and then gave himself a cultural education. There seemed to be room for an ambitious man like Pietro, a New Man for the new Italy. A joke since its protracted consolidation, Italy was finally being taken seriously by the rest of Europe. The country was an industrial force, with its own car, bicycle, and airplane manufacturers.

This period of Italy's renewal turned out to be brief, however, coming to an end with World War I. The war killed 571,000 Italian men and injured a million more. Italy itself began to fall apart. Malaria was back (the pumps in the Veneto broke down from neglect), and, with so many farmers off fighting, so was malnutrition. The countryside was on the verge of revolt. Emboldened by the revolution in Russia two years before, the Socialist party in Italy rose to challenge the country's Catholic orthodoxy. In the 1920 elections, the Socialists won a big victory, even in the conservative region of the Veneto. The voters of his town elected Pietro, just twenty-six, a council member; his fellow members nominated him to be mayor. He promised to break the entrenched power of the absentee landlords, calm the angry women who had besieged the city hall demanding food, and give the peasants what the country had promised them in return for fighting in the war: land.

Pietro proved a capable politician, playing off one faction's revolutionary enthusiasm against another's old-fashioned nationalism on the town council. He put his political capital at risk by refusing to hang the red flag outside the city hall, declaring to his fellow council members that "the tricolor—the red, white, and green flag—is the true flag of the nation." Instead of using town money to make a contribution to fight famine in Russia, as his Socialist colleagues wanted, he opened a local infant asylum and a school for illiterates.

Despite his good looks, growing power, and charisma, Pietro did not have an easy time finding a spouse. His uncle Angelo died in 1901 of a disease that to outsiders looked like lunacy; the same malady took his aunt Pierina in 1906 and his father, Giovanni, in 1913. Neighbors spoke quietly of a family tendency toward early death and insanity. Eventually, though, he met Albina, a dark, stout woman who, past thirty, was in danger of remaining a spinster for life. She was reluctant all the same, telling friends his feet were so big it would take too much wool to make him a pair of socks, but in 1920, with Pietro running for council member and Albina already pregnant, they wed. A photo from their wedding day shows Pietro, earnest and cheery, in a suit several sizes too big for him; Albina is more solemn, hair moussed, a corkscrew curl falling onto the square forehead of her mature face. Soon after, Albina gave birth to Isolina, who was followed in 1921 by Tosca (for whom Pietro would always have a special love).

Meanwhile, the situation in Italy deteriorated. The central government began to implode. Filling the vacuum, armed squads of men led by a former Socialist journalist named Benito Mussolini began taking power in the countryside. Dressed in black shirts, claiming they would restore *la razza italica* (the Italian race) to greatness, the Fascists quickly had the most powerful organization in the country, and in October 1922 they forced the king of Italy to hand power over to Mussolini.

A month later, Pietro was summoned to the impressive palazzo (the former summer home of a patrician Venetian family) that housed the town government: three men in black shirts were waiting in his office. Two were rank-and-file Fascists, the other the commissioner of the regional squadron. The commander asked pointedly whether Pietro had resigned yet. Pietro said that he had not and that he would not do so now, pointing out that only the government could ask for his resignation. The commander said he was the government now and would be happy to see Pietro gone. Pietro resisted for two weeks, at considerable personal risk, then gave in. "It is no longer possible to administer the town wisely, given the discontent that snakes through the town fomented by adversary political parties," he told the council in his farewell. The other Socialist members of the council resigned with him, turning the town's administration over to the Fascists, with whom it would remain until the end of the war.

Perhaps not surprisingly, given his conciliatory instinct, the Fascists marked Pietro for rehabilitation and admitted him into their ranks. He was never much of a party member for their side either, and when he had to put on the outfit of a Fascist, black shirt and puttees, head decorated with a Shriner's-like fez, his expression was one of embarrassment, of a man too old to be dressing like a boy.

Pietro became manager of the local agricultural cooperative. In short order, Isolina and Tosca were joined by two more sisters, Pierina in 1923 and Assunta in 1925, and then finally, after a decade of waiting, in 1931, Albina gave birth to a son, Silvano. The family found itself prospering, even as many around them were barely getting by. Pietro moved them out of the house they shared with his siblings, a house the family had occupied since the time of Vincenzo, leaving behind its low ceilings and smoky interior for the former summer residence of a Venetian patrician. There is a picture of the seven members of the family in front of their new home—Pietro, a small, well-barbered mustache under receded red hair, his belly growing as was appropriate for a *capofamiglia;* Albina, smiling now; the girls tall as saplings, in bright-collared dresses that fell to their knees; and Silvano, the baby, done up like a little gentleman, a *signorino,* in short pants with a polka-dotted ascot and a pocket square.

Pietro began to acquire businesses and property. He had leisure. He would take the train to Venice on Saturday afternoons dressed in a fur-lined cloak to attend La Fenice (Toti dal Monte, with her magnificent flutey voice, was his favorite soprano). He had plans to open a movie theater in town, too—everyone was crazy for the movies and he saw opportunity there.

But soon the course of this second war became clear. In World War I, Italy had entered the wrong war on the wrong side at the wrong time. It shed the maximum of blood for the minimum of gain and when, in 1939, Germany invaded Poland, Mussolini cast Italy's lot with Germany and Japan on the promise to fix that ratio. By 1943, it was obvious to most Italians that their country had made another huge mistake. The Americans had invaded, capturing Naples and driving up the peninsula, while the British demolished Mussolini's dream of Italian colonies in Africa. Fascism, rather than reviving the Roman empire, had undone forty years of progress. In 1943, the Italian government turned on the Fascist leader, arrested him, and tried to surrender to the Allies—only to find the Nazis, its former partners, invading from the north, occupying the part of the peninsula the Allies hadn't yet captured, and sending all the Italian men of fighting age to concentration camps.

In the Veneto, as elsewhere, there was barely contained anarchy. The Nazis had no interest in local Italian politics—they were focused on protecting Germany's southern border—so, for the next two years, until German troops in Italy surrendered in April 1945, the Nazi-controlled Italian countryside became a free-for-all where Fascists, Socialists, and Communist partisans settled scores. In the Veneto, the undeclared civil war was particularly intense. The Fascists shot or hanged partisans, and the partisans shot or hanged Fascists.

One day in the spring of 1944 Pietro opened his mail to find a threatening note. "Prepare your bones because we're going to break them soon. In the meantime, we send greetings." It was signed "Go-Sleep-with-the-Fishes." Pietro guessed that some of his old Socialist colleagues, angry about his accommodation with the Fascists, had sent it. Immediately afterward, he took to his bed with a fever. The local doctor identified the cause as an ear infection. The fever abated and Pietro tried to carry on with his work: he was the only wage earner in a house of seven.

The war had left the Veneto short of everything—meat and eggs had disappeared from the stores, and beans could only be gotten on the black market. The Fascists had boasted that Mussolini made the trains run on time, but now they weren't running at all—the Americans were bombing the rail lines and train stations and targeting ports and factories. One day a military train was machine-gunned by airplanes on the tracks behind the family house and Silvano walked out to find nothing moving as he wandered around the dead horses outside his door. The Germans billeted an officer in their house, who grew fond of the boy.

In the midst of this chaos, Pietro was not surprised to find he wasn't sleeping well. His fever came back too.* His doctor changed his diagnosis to arteriosclerosis and advised rest. The partisans had another idea. They dragged him down to the river—a tiny stream after generations of land reclamation projects—and left him there, ordering him to watch for German troops. Eventually, he made his way home.

His condition worsened. He took the train to Venice and then a boat to the hospital on the Fondamenta Nuove, but the doctors there said they would need three days to observe him and he said he didn't have the time—perhaps memories of his own father's death were beginning to come back to him. About a week later, in the middle of May 1943, he was back, accompanied by his oldest daughter, Isolina, and his wife. He stayed a week at the hospital and the visit was harrowing. Pietro was too heavy for the women to move to the bomb shelter, so they spent each night with their arms around him in his hospital room, praying, as Al-

---

* With Pietro, the story of FFI begins to take on a modern feel—not just because the methods doctors used to try to find a diagnosis for his ailment are still the current ones but because his family's response to the disease—preserved in a series of letters made available to me—was so immediate. The letter writers, especially the oldest daughter, Isolina, were excellent observers, and her descriptions of her father's condition are as accurate as any researchers have written since.

lied bombs fell from the skies and tears fell from his eyes. "*Che guerra infame,*" he said again and again, "what a miserable war." He grew confused, somnolent, and his legs began to jerk up and down. One time he got out of bed in the middle of the night and tried to open the window. "Don't you see," he said to Isolina. "Your sister Tosca's here."

Even as the bombs fell, doctors were able to run some tests. They X-rayed Pietro's spine, took fluid, and analyzed his blood and found them all normal. Stumped, they diagnosed encephalitis, inflammation of the brain, and sent him home.

Isolina and her sisters Pierina and Assunta watched the events with anxiety. Tosca was in Padua, pregnant and about to be married, eager to get home to celebrate her wedding with her family. Their mother, Albina, was afraid if Tosca heard how sick her father was she would try to make the dangerous trip, so she forbade her daughters from telling their other sister what was going on. For a while the girls complied, but after the trip to the hospital, from which Pietro had to be carried by two men to the boat, they began sneaking letters to Tosca. Assunta wrote that Pietro had a nervous system disorder with blood poisoning. "Don't worry too much," she urged, "let's hope that this passes quickly, along with all the upset of this world, and things return to normal."

Pierina was also reassuring, but Isolina, the oldest and most honest, did not see the point of lying. At the hospital the doctors had told her it was a matter of months, maybe days, and she wanted to prepare Tosca. Her tears wet the letter as she wrote it: "Papa is considerably worse than a month ago. He's lost his mind. . . . He barely speaks and when he does, he doesn't know what he's saying. When he sleeps it's even worse. He makes these little movements because his nerves are never calm. He smokes. He turns on the lights, he throws off his covers. He rubs his hands and says he has pins and needles, all this while asleep—and when he wakes up he is more tired than ever." She did not believe the hospital's diagnosis of encephalitis: her father wasn't in pain, whereas encephalitis was supposed to give you "a horrible headache."

That week the Allies bombed Marghera, an important port on the Adriatic, and Mestre, and began pounding the rail line to Trieste, which passed right by the family home—the sisters, terrified, watched from the roof, unable to move their father from the room at the top of the stairs where he lay. "Don't they have more important things to bomb than our little railway?" Assunta lamented. Even Isolina was exhausted. She could not understand how her father could be so sick and yet so lucid: "I really think by now God should say: 'Enough. You've had enough of hard things, don't you think?' " She prayed for a miracle.

A specialist came to the house soon after and said it was just a matter of time, but Assunta would not accept the verdict. Isolina was watching—and recording with almost clinical detachment—her father's symptoms: his eyes stuck open, his tongue swollen. He had a terrible cold and he seemed to be suffocating. Yet he still had moments of clarity and even joy: Isolina had put her face up to his and he'd smiled and caressed her hand. When her mother was out of earshot, she'd asked her father if he wanted to see Tosca. He recognized her name and looked up as if expecting her to walk in.

The end was coming; even Assunta couldn't deny it any longer. Pietro's stomach was swollen and he could breathe only with difficulty. On a Sunday night the family called in the priests, who drew them around their father's bedside. Pietro watched, knew, as every Catholic knows, what the moment meant. "My daughters," one priest said, "it's useless to pretend. Your father has raised you as Christians and now his job is done." As the girls tried to hold back tears, he sprinkled holy water on Pietro and said the Last Rites. *Domine non sum dignus.* After they were gone, Assunta took her father's temperature and found it was too high to measure. What was this horrible disease? she wondered. She looked into his eyes one last time and left him to her mother and Isolina. The two older women remained behind. Pietro was jerking so violently that she could hear the bed rattling in the upstairs room.

As he died, early in the morning, Isolina gave him a last kiss. "This is from Tosca," she said. In that moment Pietro turned to his wife and opened his mouth but all that came out was a piteous moan. It was June 19, 1944, and he was not quite fifty years old.

Pietro's end had come more quickly than anyone expected. A group of cousins on their way to see him from another part of the Veneto arrived on their bicycles to find a casket. Silvano, barely a teenager, hid upstairs as family and friends filled the family room where his father lay. Three days later, the funeral mass was held, Albina and the five children surrounded by hundreds of mourners. Assunta tried hard to accept God's verdict: "His will was done," she kept saying to herself. Her *papà* was now in heaven. Isolina drew a harsher lesson: God had not found her worthy. After the mass, her grief reached almost biblical proportions. She climbed up onto the hearse and rode to the cemetery burning with love for the father she had lost. He had accompanied her on her wedding day dressed in white, she thought, and now it was her turn to accompany him dressed in black. Everyone admired her courage.

Pietro was buried next to his uncle Michele in a plot in the cemetery he'd bought when he was mayor. The funeral cost five thousand lire, an enormous amount of money. How, the girls worried, were they going to survive without their father? He had been waiting until Silvano grew up to bring him into the family business. Now they would be reduced to poverty.

Meanwhile, the Allies had landed at Normandy and captured Rome. The war would soon be over: a new era was beginning, but the family was too devastated to notice.

Of course, the hospital that misdiagnosed Pietro's illness had no idea what prion diseases were or what they might look like. But had the staff looked harder, they might have found two recent entries in the catalogue of neurological diseases that would have set them on the right path: Creutzfeldt-Jakob disease and Gerstmann-Sträussler-Scheinker disease.

In the 1910s, a German doctor named Hans Creutzfeldt saw a twenty-three-year-old patient named Berta. Berta's disease at first looked like pellagra—she had dementia and her skin was red—but pellagra had basically been eliminated from Europe by then. Over time, Berta lost the ability to walk, and she began to shake. She screamed as if possessed, claimed she was a murderer, and then laughed uncontrollably. She grew feverish, then slipped into a coma and died. Creutzfeldt decided to examine her brain.

The Italians had once been the best anatomists, then the French, but by the late nineteenth century, the Germans were preeminent. They were superb theorists and had the best tissue staining and preservation techniques. Even German doctors, though, were divided over whether it was worth the trouble to autopsy a brain—it was a black box whose mix of neurons and tissues seemed unlikely to explain the complexities of the human mind. "Anatomy," the psychiatrist Emil Kraepelin said, "can contribute nothing to psychiatry." Creutzfeldt disagreed. He sectioned Berta's brain, mounted it on slides, and examined it. He saw dead neurons everywhere, a surprise because neurological diseases with her symptoms typically had very narrow, concentrated decay. He did not know what to make of what he saw, and after World War I he published his observations.

Creutzfeldt's paper would have been forgotten if not for another German neurologist, Alfons Maria Jakob, who read it after examining a series of middle-aged men and women in his own lab in Munich a decade later. The symptoms of his patients, some of whom were related, were similar to those Creutzfeldt saw in Berta: they too lost the ability to walk; their limbs jerked; they were disoriented and became demented before dying. He suggested that he and Creutzfeldt had been looking at the same disease. Several years after, another neurologist reviewing Jakob's work christened the disease "Jakob-Creutzfeldt disease."

Another piece of the prion disease mystery fell into place shortly after, in 1928 in Vienna, where a neurologist named Josef Gerstmann treated a twenty-six-year-old woman. She walked clumsily, and every time she turned her head her arms crossed. By 1936, Gerstmann, along with two other researchers, Ernst Sträussler and I. Mark Scheinker, had gathered together a small group of patients with similar symptoms. They tended to be older than Gerstmann's first patient and their overall symptoms were less peculiar, but they too experienced memory loss and poor coordination and, sometimes, dementia. Several of the sufferers were related. On autopsy, the victims were found to have plaques in the brain, which reminded the Viennese neurologists of Alzheimer's disease, but missing were the regions of dead cells and astrocytes—star-shaped cells, a sign of attempted neuron regrowth after trauma—that Jakob had seen in his patients.

Had the Venetian doctors been aware of any of this work, or had they thought to look at the charts for Pietro's brother Luigi, who had died in the same Venice hospital fourteen years before him, they would have had the beginnings of a diagnosis—an established pathology that appeared inheritable. They might also have found illuminating an observation made by the German researchers that conventional lab studies (such as those done in Venice on Pietro) did not reveal any irregularities. There was no evidence of infection in the spinal fluid or the blood of sufferers and nothing striking in the pathology of the brain, at least to the naked eye. But when the neurologist examined sections of the victims' brains under a microscope, they saw that the brains were badly damaged—full of holes, astrocytes, and plaques, piles of tangled dead protein.

Pietro's siblings died of FFI in steady succession: Angela in 1948,

Maria in 1957, Emma in 1965, and Irma in 1966. From the point of view of medical knowledge, it was as if they never lived. Not that a diagnosis linking their disease to Jakob-Creutzfeldt disease or Gerstmann-Sträussler-Scheinker disease would have meant much. After a spate of efforts in the 1920s, interest in the conditions died down. Every year or two, a case of one or the other would appear in the medical literature and elicit only a shrug from neurologists. By 1968 there were still only 150 CJD victims on the books. Such scarcity made researchers wonder whether CJD was a discrete disease at all. Maybe, a group of British neurologists posited in a 1968 book, it was nothing "more than a convenient dumping ground for otherwise unclassifiable dementias with interesting cross relations to certain systemic deteriorations." A refutation of this position would only start to come fifteen years after Pietro's death, and half a world away.

PART II

PUSHING BACK THE DARK

CHAPTER 4

STRONG MAGIC PAPUA NEW GUINEA, *1947*

Young man, be careful! I ate your grandfather.

—ELDERLY FORE to his nurse at an Okapa hospital

The Fore were a primitive tribe on the island of Papua New Guinea. In the late 1950s Western doctors found they were suffering from a mysterious ailment called kuru, which, they discovered, was related to scrapie. The scientists trying to understand the outbreak had tools that nineteenth-century scrapie investigators like Baron von Richthofen and Roche-Lubin could not have dreamed of. They had electron microscopes and X-ray crystallography. They could see viruses and determine the structure of proteins almost down to the atom. They knew that DNA made RNA, which in turn made the body's thousands of proteins, and that these proteins consisted mostly of amino acids bound together according to the laws of physics.

Yet all this new knowledge had a downside: it made scientists less flexible about exceptions to the two rules it had taken them such work to acquire in the previous decades, 1) that genes determine the characteristics of living things, and 2) that only living things cause infection. It made it harder to see when these laws weren't true. How did you make the leap to understand something that shouldn't exist: a nonliving molecule that reproduced itself and caused an infection as if it were living? It would take a researcher as visionary as Carleton Gajdusek, who in 1976 won a Nobel Prize for his work, to start to answer that question.

In 1918, as a reward for being on the winning side of World War I, the League of Nations gave Australia control of the eastern half of New Guinea, formerly a German possession. This reward turned out to be as much a burden as a blessing. A great deal of blood had been spilled over the previous 350 years as Europeans tried to get a foothold on the coasts of the island. Malaria and combative cannibalistic natives made every settlement a battlefield. During this time, Europeans believed that the interior of the island was empty. There was no evidence that anyone lived in New Guinea's mountainous interior under its vast rainforest canopy.

Then came the airplane, and the Australians learned that there were many hundreds of thousands of people in the interior—people who in their eyes weren't much friendlier than the coastal natives had been. They were in a state of perpetual conflict with each other, bows and arrows and stone axes at the ready, with a willingness to use them on passersby. Many of the Highland tribes turned out to be cannibals too—at least, that was the word the Australians got.

But the Australians, having settled their own continent, were looking for adventure. There was money to be made in the Highlands— gold, timber, and coffee money—and heathen souls to be saved. These reasons, though, were subsidiary to the deepest one for entering the region. What the Australians wanted—as they told themselves and foreigners again and again—was not to conquer the Highlanders but to "contact" them. The goal was to tap the natives on their shoulders and introduce them to the wonders of the modern world: radios and telephones; penicillin; disease-resistant modern grains and tractors with which to plant them. The Australians wanted to bring them good news.

So in the 1940s Australia pulled together a team of officials to send into the Highlands. It is significant that the patrol officers, as they were known, were not trained to use firearms. They carried rifles, but their most important weapons were their notebooks. Their job was to observe, pacify when necessary, and foremost, to report. What they wrote was read by their supervisors in Port Moresby, the island capital, and then mimeo'ed and sent to Canberra, whence the Australians administered their new protectorate.

The patrol officers had a difficult task. The highlands were a patchwork of hundreds of tribes—the Kukukuku (now called the Anga),* the Kamano, the Awa—each occupying only a few square miles and comprising between several hundred and several thousand members. More than three hundred languages were spoken in a tiny area. The patrol officer was supposed to travel from village to village through this crazy quilt, conducting a census and providing basic medical care. Native policemen from the coast would accompany him on his trip, along with porters hauling crates of shells and metal axes for trade.

It wasn't until 1947 that patrol officers reached the small tracts of nearly vertical rain forest to the south of the Kratke Mountains between the Lamari and the Yani rivers. This area was among the last territories to be "contacted," and it was there that Australia's patrol officers had their first encounter with the Fore. One day R. I. Skinner, an army veteran who was an exception to the patrol officer culture in that he often patrolled with a machine gun, showed up in the Fore territory and fired some rounds into the ground. The tribe, terrified,

---

* Today, "Kukukuku" is a derogatory term. "Anga" is the preferred term. I have kept the outdated (and now offensive) usage where historically appropriate.

thought he was some sort of divine being. They began ritual purifications. The men played their sacred flutes and refrained from intercourse with their women.

The Fore's fear and confusion were understandable; countless centuries of development separated them from this intruder. Skinner wore cotton woven into cloth by a machine and shaved with steel. The Fore dressed in grass skirts and had feathers in their hair, and the men wore penis shields made of bird bone. They used no money and had no written language. In fact, they had no name for themselves ("Fore," pronounced *For*-ay, was what their neighbors called them. It meant "down there" or "to the south"). They had no idea they lived on an island, or even what an island was.

The Fore had a subsistence economy. They lived on sweet potato and taro root, supplementing their garden vegetables with game the men hunted. The women and children captured rats and bugs by hand and ate them. The Fore kept pigs as well, whose foraging they tried to control: much of the men's work consisted of fencing the gardens against animals. Pigs were enormously valuable and prestigious possessions, so they lived with the women in their huts, where sometimes they were suckled ahead of Fore babies.

When the Fore weren't growing food or hunting it, they often were fighting. They lived in fortified hamlets, and the cause of a skirmish might be an offense against oneself, one's wife, one's pigs, or one's garden. The battles were small but lethal and constant: a dozen men would lay siege to a hamlet. They threw their spears, fired off their arrows, then retreated to wait behind the stockades that surrounded their homes for the inevitable counterattack. The Fore had good aim. Violence was the leading cause of death among their men, others of whom had only one eye left. War never decided anything permanently; that was not its purpose. The combatants were usually linked either by marriage or through reciprocal obligations and the skirmish was one more entry in an endless tally of favors and grievances by which the social hierarchy was established. Alliances came and went, and the members of a hamlet that had attacked another might be found at their opponents' next pig feast.

The Australians expected to be one more feuding party in this Hobbesian state of affairs. This was what previous "first contact" had brought them. But not with this tribe. As the patrol officers entered each town, the Fore laid down their arms and lined up to be counted. In Lufa, for instance, on July 5, 1951, a patrol officer named A. T. Carey, known as "Tiny," recorded, "The natives received us very enthusiastically. To my knowledge this was the first time that a patrol had remained more than a few hours, and this was very evident in their reception of us. Suffice it to say they were very pleased."

Carey, in his early twenties, was an exceptional patrol officer, as was his colleague John McArthur, whose sympathy for native life some patrol officers mocked by nicknaming him John Kukukuku. Both were suspicious that the tribe's cooperation was just for show; they wondered what was really going on. But the warm receptions continued. Soon the Fore were building rest houses and patrol posts for the Australians. All they seemed to want in return were the census books.

Shortly after the patrol officers' arrival, the Fore gave up war, they gave up the men's hut and the initiation rituals that went on in it, they surrendered their sacred flutes. They replaced some of their sweet potato and taro crops with the cash crop of coffee. They opened trading stores. They signed up to work on Australian projects on the coast. They abandoned their enormously complex culture. They even gave up the custom they said they had of eating their dead.

In fact, things seemed to be changing so fast the Australians tried to slow the process down. Too-rapid assimilation could undermine the hierarchy between Australian and native. The Australians didn't understand that the people they were trying to preserve as primitive were, in a deeper way, their counterparts. Australia was a self-invented country of settlers. The Fore, too, were a can-do frontier people, who didn't care at all who their ancestors were or what social position they held. They were innovators, makers and molders of their own selves.

The first contact with the Fore was a surprise, a nearly entirely happy one from the Australian point of view. The most perceptive patrol officers, though, still suspected they weren't seeing the whole picture. They wondered whether the Fore were leading double lives, and they looked for evidence to confirm the suspicion. There must be a secret somewhere; why would a primitive people give up their culture this fast? Over time the officers noticed they weren't seeing very many sick people or, for that matter, many women. Many primitive tribes had the custom of sequestering their women from European eyes; maybe the Fore did too. But that did not explain, as John McArthur noted, the number of unmarried young men in the Fore hamlets.

The mystery of the latrines came next. Since first contact, patrol officers had regularly instructed the Fore in the need to dig toilets, but this was a Western custom that the Fore had mostly ignored. They were a casual people, casual about food, sex, and child-rearing. When dealing with excretion, the Fore just used the bushes, to the disgust and concern of the patrol officers. Then, the Fore started digging latrines. It didn't make sense. At first the latrine digging took place mostly in the north, which was more culturally sophisticated, while in the south the toilets remained "mostly rude and rough, being sometimes merely a hole in the ground," as McArthur noted. But soon the Southerners were digging proper toilets too. With each visit from the patrols, the Fore seemed to throw themselves into the effort with more energy.

"Tiny" Carey noted something in the middle of August 1950 that deepened this mystery. He noticed that near the village of Henganofi there had been an unusual number of deaths. "It appears," he wrote his superiors, "natives suffer from stomach trouble, get violent shivering, as with the ague, and die fairly rapidly." He had sent the cases on to Goroka, the regional capital, adding that among the natives " 'poison' has been mooted as the reason." McArthur investigated a little more. He was running a new patrol post in the local capital of Okapa, where his primary job was to dynamite a route for a road to Goroka, opening up the region for ordinary transport and work—and, not incidentally, reminding the Fore of the power behind the white man's notebooks. One day in August 1953 he ran into more of the shivering people Tiny Carey had seen several years before: "Nearing one of the dwellings, I observed a small girl sitting down beside a fire. She was shivering violently and her head was jerking spasmodically from side to side."

The locals explained that she was "a victim of sorcery and would continue thus, shivering and unable to eat, until death claimed her within a few weeks," he wrote. Sorcery played an important role in the lives of the Fore, who were particularly feared by their neighbors for their knowledge of the black arts. Sorcery served to explain nearly everything they could not explain through visible cause and effect. The Fore used it to account for nearly all deaths other than those in war—as well as for how the white man's rifles worked and where the Australians got the materials with which they made their airplanes and their penicillin.

The Fore called the sorcery that afflicted the shivering women kuru ("shaking"). Kuru was particularly easy to inflict. All one needed was a bundle made up of leaves and a bit of the potential victim's effects: clothes, hair, or feces. The bundle was then buried and when the evildoer wanted the victim to shiver, he dug it up and gave it a shake. Kuru was also easy to forestall: all the victim had to do was find the bundle and destroy it. But prevention was the best medicine against kuru: the smartest thing was to put your personal effects where no one could get at them. That's why the Fore had been digging such deep latrine holes (a patrol officer described one as "bottomless"): so that no one could get down them to retrieve their excrement.

The patrol officers decided to put a stop to the hysteria that they were sure was causing the strange outbreak. John McArthur ordered the Fore to bring their antisorcery implements to a big bonfire. The tribe complied. Then he threatened with arrest the next person who claimed countersorcery skills. Soon after, John Colman, a patrol officer who succeeded McArthur, stood up in front of the Fore and put a sorcery bundle in his mouth to show how harmless it was (then he discreetly spat it out).

But the deaths from shaking increased. The Australians began to realize that a doctor had to be sent for to see what was really going on. So in 1955, the department of health in Moresby assigned Vincent Zigas to the Eastern Highlands. For most doctors, such a posting would have been a punishment. But not for the Lithuanian-born Zigas. Deeply scarred by the Second World War, during which he said he had worked as a doctor on the German side, he fell in love with unspoiled New Guinea. As Carleton Gajdusek, who would later team up with him, noted, Zigas felt the "romanticism of the Central European for the Black Man and his lands." His "somewhat mopish mood," Zigas wrote in one of two memoirs he published, was "enlivened" by the Fore, these "martial people" whose dignity was so unlike his own situation among the Australians, where, because he was foreign born, he was just a "bloody Wog."

The Highlands offered Zigas a challenge without degradation, but little else. There were no surgical facilities; even sterilizing a wound was hard. And the Fore were still skeptical of Western medicine. One day one of Zigas's native nurses was trying to get an older patient to cooperate. As in many cultures, the elderly were accustomed to more respect. "Young man, be careful!" the old man warned him. "I ate your grandfather."

Zigas's two highly embellished memoirs are full of lambent moonlight and all-night native feasts. In them, he recounts first hearing about kuru shortly after taking up his posting, at a bar in Kainantu, where he overheard John McArthur holding forth on his region and its problems. Zigas introduced himself. McArthur asked if he'd seen his 1953 report on the bewitched girl shivering by the fire. When Zigas said no, McArthur, five rums in him, began wildly cursing the Port Moresby bureaucrats who were sitting on the information. Two months later, McArthur sent a note with a Fore man named Apekono, who was there to take Zigas to see the strange disease. The note, wrapped in an envelope of breadfruit leaves tied with jungle vine, read "Follow Apekono. Stop. Be my Bunkie, no tucker needed. Stop. Grog and penicillin appreciated." It was signed "John Blotto." "Bunkie" was a housemate. "Tucker" was food. "Grog," of course, was liquor. Blotto was McArthur.

Travel in the Fore part of the Highlands was hard. One walked on tiny, irregular paths, following native guides. It took Apekono four days to take Zigas the fifty miles to the village of Moke, where McArthur was patrolling. On the way, Apekono stopped at a hut and showed Zigas his first kuru victim. "On the ground in the far corner sat a woman of about thirty," the doctor wrote. "She looked odd, not ill, rather emaciated, looking up with blank eyes with a mask-like expression. There was an occasional fine tremor of her head and trunk, as if she were shivering from cold, though the day was very warm." It was almost exactly the tableau McArthur had witnessed in 1953. Zigas, though, was a doctor. He could do more than look—or so he thought: "I decided I might as well try my own variety of magic," he remembered. He rubbed Sloan's Liniment, a balm for sore muscles, on her and declared to her family and his guide: "The sorcerer has put a bad spirit inside the woman. I am going to burn this spirit so that it comes out of her and leaves her. You will not see the fire, but she will feel it. The bad spirit will leave her and she will not die."

The lotion penetrated the woman's skin and she writhed in pain. "Get up! Walk!" Zigas commanded theatrically. "The woman struggled feebly as if to rise, then, exhausted, started to tremble more violently, making a sound of foolish laughter, akin to a titter." That evening Apekono asked Zigas not to try to cure any more kuru victims; "Don't use your magic medicine anymore. It will not win our strong sorcery."

There was the point. If Fore magic was seen as stronger than European magic, the Australians' whole colonial adventure would collapse. Prestige was of incalculable importance in the Highlands, where a few hundred Europeans dominated hundreds of thousands of Highlanders, and the Australians' inability to stop the spread of kuru was beginning to injure their standing in the eyes of the natives. As the deaths continued, the Fore grew less and less willing to line up for censuses or submit to the administrative proceedings by which the Australians enforced their law. They developed what one patrol officer called "an attitude of intense dislike and passive resistance towards the Administration."

Then a cargo cult began. It was one of the first in the Fore region. Cargo cults were mystical movements that promised natives a share in the affluence of the whites. The members of a cargo cult built a special house, which they sealed, and each day, they prayed for the arrival within the house of European goods—canned foods, ammunition, clothes. Inevitably, when they opened the door of the house, they were disappointed and angry, wondering why the colonists' magic did not work for them too. Cargo cults were a sign of societal strain, of a loss of faith in European promises.

Jack Baker, a patrol officer who followed McArthur and Colman, confiscated the charm of the leaders of the cargo cult and hoped the anger would die down. But kuru was by now responsible for half the deaths in the district, six hundred deaths in the previous five years by Baker's count. Until that changed, kuru-afflicted villages were going to be agitated ones.

Vincent Zigas considered the symptoms of kuru. The victims shivered in the heat. They grew glassy-eyed and cross-eyed. They lost their sense of balance. Some kuru sufferers walked clumsily or kept falling down. Others seemed fine except for the trembling of the hands that seemed the first symptom of the disease. Many sick Fore, when Zigas questioned them about their condition, giggled or laughed in an anxious, involuntary response. He learned to tell future kuru victims by the strange way they held their heads.

Zigas wanted to know what was causing the condition. So he sent blood samples to the head health officer at Port Moresby. When Port Moresby was stumped, he sent serum samples and even a brain that he persuaded a victim's family to part with to the Hall Institute in Melbourne, the best laboratory in Australia. There, Dr. Gray Anderson, a capable virologist, looked for evidence of virus or bacteria, without success. Whatever kuru was, it didn't cause its victims to make antibodies in response.

There was more confusing information. Zigas kept running into kuru sufferers who said they had recovered. Were there, then, two kurus, one real and one false? To Zigas, a disease that could be turned on again and off again and yielded only negative lab results suggested that the Fore were the victims of group hysteria.

The Fore, however, had no problem understanding their situation. They knew kuru was both a real physical disease and a product of sorcery, and they were comfortable with its dual reality. This was not because they did not believe in infection. They did—they knew infection came quickly and to people who gathered together, sharing food and drink. Infection could change a whole hamlet from well to sick in a day or a week. But kuru didn't spread that way. It attacked women and children far more often than men, killing whole families except the husband. It also appeared to affect women who had left the hamlet to marry outsiders years earlier. That pattern reinforced the Fores' certainty that sorcery was responsible: women were very valuable in the Fore world and men paid high bride prices for them. A person who killed your wife was committing a kind of theft.

What didn't make sense to the Fore, though, was the enormous number of deaths. The Fore were always at war, but they would never go so far as to depopulate a town or a region. All those one-eyed men were a telling indication of restraint: Poke out two eyes and a man was useless; take out one eye and he had simply been warned.

Eventually, however, the Fore traced the beginning of the kuru epidemic to their satisfaction. Years before, a frustrated suitor had a woman killed to punish her brothers, who had refused permission for their marriage. This affront had begun the kuru war. For a while, the Fore tried to tamp down the battle through a technique called *tukabu,* in which the relatives of a kuru victim caught the sorcerer, bashed in his head with stones, and crushed his genitals. But this was not sufficient to stop the kuru deaths. The women began to object; why weren't the men stopping the kuru that led to so much misery among their number? They pointed out that by hexing so many women, the men were digging their own graves: "Try to find one man who is pregnant now and show him to us," they demanded. And a young man said, "Look at the bush growing up around us where we once had lines of people working in their gardens. Soon there will be no one here to look after it." Indeed, bride prices were skyrocketing, men were going without wives, and pigs were not getting the care they needed, either, as the men took the place of the dead (and never born) women who had worked the gardens.

Fore leaders, called "big men," held meetings to discuss the problem. In one gathering, the sorcerers in their midst were asked to identify themselves. Man after man admitted his transgression. Then he put the offending hand in water and promised not to practice sorcery again. Every man, it turned out, had played a role. Repentance held the promise of a break in the cycle of hex-reprisal-hex. Balance would be restored, the invisible hand fixed.

But even before these events, the Australians watched the impact of kuru with great concern. They had hoped to teach the European countries a lesson in how to modernize a Stone Age people. Instead, their charges were mysteriously dying of a disease that might just be a hysterical reaction to the very societal changes the Australians had expected to be welcomed for. Dr. Zigas was stumped, and his superiors in the government had no clue what to do next, either.

CHAPTER 5

DOCTA AMERICA PAPUA NEW GUINEA, *1957*

This strange white bloke would appear out of the bush, jabber at you in a language you didn't understand, stick a needle into you, write something in a book, and then move on.

—NEW GUINEA PATROL OFFICER describing a
visit from Carleton Gajdusek

On the morning of March 8, 1957, thirty-three-year-old Carleton Gajdusek found himself in the office of the acting head of the department of public health in Port Moresby, New Guinea. Gajdusek was a complicated and controversial man, a brilliant researcher and pediatrician, who took an intense sexualized interest in the children he studied. Born in Yonkers, New York, to a middle-class family, he never had any doubt what he wanted to grow up to be. His favorite book in childhood was Paul de Kruif's *The Microbe Hunters,* a romanticized chronicle of researchers like Pasteur and Koch who solved the mysteries of medicine. He and his brother wrote the great names of medicine on the wall of the staircase leading to their attic workroom.

Gajdusek went to the University of Rochester, where he studied biophysics, and then on to Harvard Medical School. He did a postdoctorate in physical chemistry at the California Institute of Technology under Linus Pauling (he told his friend Gunther Stent he was there to straighten out Pauling's ideas about proteins), and also studied with the founder of molecular biology, Max Delbrück. He did additional work on microbiology at Harvard with the famous John Enders, often thought of as the father of American virology. All three of his teachers would win Nobel Prizes.

In the early 1950s, as an army doctor, Gajdusek helped trace the cause of a hemorrhagic fever that was killing American soldiers in Korea to migratory birds. In 1954, the Centers for Disease Control sent him on a secret mission to Bolivia to investigate an apparent epidemic among a group of Okinawans whom the U.S. Navy had transported to South America after World War II. There were rumors that the United States was running concentration camps. Gajdusek was able to attribute the deaths to natural causes—if "natural causes" included death by arrow wound—and the CDC was impressed enough to offer him a job: "You're a screwball," his supervisor said, "but you're my kind of screwball." Gajdusek declined the offer. Instead he arranged to study with Sir Macfarlane Burnet (known as "Sir Mac") of the Hall Institute in Melbourne, himself on the way to a Nobel Prize for his work on acquired immunological tolerance.

Gajdusek had learned bench science from the best. But he was also keenly interested in practical medicine—in curing the sick, especially sick children. He had turned down offers to move into more theoretical research, and he wrote in the voluminous journal he kept: "In the slow routine of buffer preparation, microscope peering, egg inoculating and chick embryo lung harvesting, where does the challenge of the intellectual endeavor lie? . . . I often wonder whether there is not

more abstract thought and intellectual curiosity and deductive and in-
ductive reasoning involved at the bedside of a sick child." This was not
just pretense: the health of children mattered to Gajdusek.

Gajdusek had chosen Port Moresby as the entry point for a grandly
conceived, multinational study of "child growth, development and behavior and disease patterns in primitive and isolated cultures" that he
had set up to follow his fellowship with Sir Mac. In typical fashion, he
had arranged the tour by himself; he would worry about academic
sponsors later. From Port Moresby he would head to Lufa, a village in
the Highlands where Ian Burnet, Sir Mac's son, was working as a patrol officer, and after New Guinea, he would visit other islands in the
region. Some of these territories had yet to be controlled, so to enter
them he needed permission of the government: whence his appearance in Port Moresby.

Port Moresby was not Gajdusek's kind of town. It was much too civ-
ilized, and in exactly the way he detested. It was full of tea parties and
gossip, and he suspected there was a degenerate side the town was
ashamed to acknowledge. He switched from a nice hotel to a cheaper,
more real one at "two guineas a day." Even there the waiters and cab-
bies and other young men ignored this odd-looking white man with his
thatch of hair and thick black glasses. "The whole setting mediates
against any real friendship or close association," he complained in his
journal.

To Gajdusek's mind, Port Moresby was a perfect example of what he
saw as the problem of the West: it smashed the individual. Earlier, on a
Sunday in Melbourne, he had gone into the city while the residents
worshipped in church. He noted in his diary, "I pray—and I would
plead to the Christ, if I could believe, knowing that he would understand and heed—that these youths may yet enjoy their days of the flesh
in flagrant 'sinning' before it is too late . . . for only then will they have
lived." And in Sydney he looked at the water and thought how the surf
was more alive "than its inhabitants who are passively tossed in it. Few

master this surf!" He was eager to master the surf himself, and this tour of Oceania was meant, as much as anything, to find where the waves were breaking—to do important work in medicine and to satisfy his unconventional sexual impulses. He guessed his destination would be a wild place, not a tame one, and he hoped it would be with children, in part because his medical specialty was pediatrics. His pedophilia, he later claimed, had been with him since his childhood.

But Gajdusek's early writings suggest more uncertainty than courage in putting his sexual proclivities into action. His journals of the time contain pathetic accounts of semiarticulated attraction. For all his desire to master the surf, he hesitates. "Little to write of—little of moment. I live poised for a sudden movement . . . but do not dare to take it," he writes in February 1956, sounding more like J. Alfred Prufrock than a fearless wanderer.

During these self-appointed rounds Gajdusek was discontented, still looking for an important problem to solve. "Joe," he wrote to Joseph Smadel, his chief supporter at the National Institutes of Health, almost six months before he found kuru, "I frankly am shopping and trying to find a place to continue work. . . . If you have any opportunities wherein I can fit . . . and you know well what a recalcitrant and unpredictable subordinate I make . . . I shall be most interested and grateful." Smadel, who had supervised Gajdusek at the Walter Reed Army Institute of Research in Washington, did not suggest a new office job. He knew that Gajdusek needed the field, where he might make significant discoveries and find romance. He was aware, too, that Gajdusek was as much an ethnographer as a scientist; it was a tendency Smadel was constantly trying to tamp down. "When you go over this," Smadel wrote to him in 1956, enclosing one of the half dozen papers Gajdusek was working on at the time, "do not add the innumerable conversationally interesting points. . . . Furthermore, do not ask for us to include any travelogue pictures in this paper, so what if they live in mud houses or holes in the ground. Remember the old dictum in newspaper writing—if you are in doubt about the pertinence of a paragraph, leave it out."

But Gajdusek could not possibly respect that request. His secret life, his adolescent imagination, and his intense curiosity always rebelled against limits. What interested him was what was marginal, coincidental, picturesque. When he traveled, he sometimes concocted a background: he was the son of a wealthy socialite who had educated him by traveling through Europe. Besides his wanderlust, another manifestation of Gajdusek's rebellion against limits was his logorrhea—he had already written ten volumes of diaries in imitation of André Gide.

What Gajdusek learned when he talked to Dr. R.F.R. Scragg, the acting director of the Papua New Guinea department of health in Port Moresby, changed his life. A balding career public health doctor who had recently been promoted, Scragg was by nature an organization man. He assumed that Gajdusek, as Gajdusek remembered, was "Sir Mac's man" in Port Moresby. So he gave the American a file detailing everything in which the institute was involved in Papua New Guinea.

Gajdusek read in the file about an intriguing medical mystery that was unfolding among the Fore of the Eastern Highlands.

Sir Mac was tired of Australian medicine living in the shadow of English and American medicine, and in kuru he had seen an opportunity to redress that. Handsome and charismatic, Sir Mac was a major presence in his home country and had the power, unlike the "bloody Wog" Vincent Zigas, to convince the government to throw resources at the kuru epidemic. His first step, in early 1957, had been to arrange to send Gray Anderson, the virologist who had looked at the kuru tissue that Zigas had sent the Hall Institute, to Okapa, in the Highlands, to look around.

Now, seeing the papers that contained the evidence of Sir Mac's deviousness, Gajdusek was angry. Sir Mac had known about the disease; he in fact had already received a brain with kuru to study! Gajdusek was supposedly his protégé. Wasn't he even now on his way to visit his son? Yet Sir Mac had told him nothing about kuru. Gajdusek wrote in his diary: "Bitter? No? Just disappointed at my fallen idol . . . for my, how he falls!!!"

Gajdusek realized that he had arrived in New Guinea just in time. Sir Mac's virologist Anderson ought already to have been in the Highlands looking at kuru—if it hadn't been for his wife: she had demanded to know what the safeguards were against "possible dangers from hostile native reaction" against her husband. What sort of life insurance would the Andersons have? She had asked her husband, who had asked Sir Mac, who had cabled Scragg, who had kicked the query upstairs to his boss, who was waiting for an answer to "allay any fears Mrs. Anderson may have."

So while Anderson was waiting for news of his death benefit, Gajdusek, who had no wife and no fears—he told everyone he hoped to be dead by forty—simply booked a flight to Goroka via Wau on the Papua side of the border. Five days later he was in Kainantu, the district capital closest to kuru country. Immediately he was in love with the Highlands. He met Zigas and liked him. Zigas was lively, a character—one patrol officer remembered him as "Danny Kaye playing a middle-European doctor." Indeed, many who worked with him, including Gajdusek, even wondered whether Zigas really had a medical degree. The two hit it off: Zigas was willing to work hard and give Gajdusek the glory, while Gajdusek could cheer up the "mopish" Zigas. He could inspire Zigas to do what he should have been doing all along: throwing all his energy into the problem of kuru.

Cables were now flying back and forth from Sir Mac to Scragg in Port Moresby, to his superiors in Canberra, to Anderson, still waiting in the wings in Melbourne, to Sir Mac again. Gajdusek had double-crossed his hosts, he was in kuru country illegally, and he was told to leave without delay. Sir Mac worried about what Scragg called "another American invasion." He could feel a chance for a major discovery slipping away from Australian medicine. But Gajdusek wasn't going anywhere: he had before him an isolated tribe, in the Fore; a willing subordinate, in Zigas; and preteens who had not been exposed to the West's paralyzing morality. The stories that the Fore had until recently practiced ritual cannibalism, eating the bodies of their dead as a tribute (and some said the custom continued, just out of sight of Westerners), thrilled Gajdusek too. "Women and children, particularly, partake of the human flesh," he noted with pleasure. An hour after meeting Zigas, he wrote to the Australians that "[Zigas] tells me that all (yes, astoundingly, all 100%) of 28 cases collected two to four months ago are now dead!" He had found the best medical problem of the decade.

Gajdusek made the Australians an offer: They would consult on the investigation. He would do the dirty work of bushwhacking with a bunch of savages, keeping Sir Mac "informed of our every move." He even promised them a fresh kuru brain to dissect. In the meantime, to hold off Scragg, the man who'd first told him about kuru and was trying to throw him out, he found an excuse to stay: he had run into some infants with upper-respiratory ailments among the Fore. "Intensive investigation uninterruptible," Gajdusek cabled. "Will remain at work with patients to whom we are responsible. Am in direct correspondence with Sir Mac." Sure enough, Sir Mac, who was not immune to Gajdusek's charm and energy (and, besides, knew when he had been beaten), fell in line. Anderson, he decided, could study Murray Valley encephalitis instead; Gajdusek would get kuru.

Gajdusek's approach to kuru was to try everything and try it quickly, no matter what the obstacle—interview, bleed, preserve, ship the blood, analyze the lab results—then move to the next hamlet and do the same.

"We are lab minded," he wrote to Scragg, asking for more supplies. And numbers minded. By early April 1957, he had thirteen new active cases and records of as many deaths. That made forty-one in total, nearly half of whom were children. By mid-May he had almost seventy active cases. Thirty more suspected cases appeared by the end of the month, and every one was dying. By the end of June, Gajdusek and Zigas had records of two hundred deaths. The female–male mortality ratio in adults now appeared to be over fourteen-to-one, and the symptoms of the sufferers could not have been odder: victims stumbled, they grew cross-eyed, they became "belligerent or aggressive." Gajdusek noted their "emotional instability" and "tendency to excessive hilarity," their "euphoric grins and smiles, or even shrieks." He wrote Smadel, "Could any more astounding and remarkable picture be found anywhere?" Smadel found Gajdusek a grant and sent him a camera and film to make movies of what he saw and scientific papers and instructions as he requested them.

As he had promised, Gajdusek sent his furious Australian hosts a brain. At the same time he sent brains to Smadel at the NIH. It was a difficult balancing act, pleasing and courting both parties, and the whole thing had just the madcap tone that Gajdusek loved. One time he sent Sir Mac the brain of a patient and Smadel the viscera. Gajdusek managed to separate ten more kuru victims from their brains and grew confident there would be enough tissue for everyone. He did many of the extractions on his dinner table, sometimes using a carving knife (his father was a butcher), storing the tissue in the camp refrigerator. Some relatives of some kuru victims were squeamish. Gajdusek would give them tins of food, salt, or lap-laps (native skirts) as gifts to obtain their consent.

Gajdusek's first goal was to figure out what type of disease kuru was—genetic, infectious, environmental, or psychosomatic. While he waited for labs in the United States and Melbourne to give him answers, he undertook his epidemiological investigation. He investigated everything the Fore ate, drank, or touched. He suspected the smoke in their huts and the copper in their water. He saw that manioc, a local vegetable, could be toxic if it wasn't handled carefully. He moved through the bush with Zigas, the patrol officer Jack Baker, and Jack's dog, Kuru. Gajdusek, Baker remembered, would bring boxes of crayons and get the children of the hamlet drawing, then ask them questions, a Pied Piper.

Gajdusek's interest in children served the Fore well. "They used him medically," Baker remembered. "I saw him nursing sick children back to life, almost willing them." In turn, the Fore told him about kuru. The "detailed epidemiology" grew to one thousand cards, an unheard-of abundance—neurology was a field in which any doctor would be lucky to see a half dozen cases of a given disease in a lifetime.

Kuru was a puzzle, like the paths Gajdusek trod through the bush. Did the disease run in families; or did it cluster in hamlets? Did people contract the disease in the same place at the same time? Or at the same place at different times? Had anyone ever gone into remission from kuru? What was the role of hysteria in the disease? Gajdusek set up a Kuru Research Post in Okapa, built with the help of a thousand natives. From there he sent live patients to Moresby and then to Australia for EEGs to look for "petit mal triad-type records," a sign of epilepsy, or "anything resembling the slow wave–high blocated pattern of post-encephalitis." He considered everything: Sydenham's chorea, Wilson's disease, African sleeping sickness, "fatal anoerexia nervosa plus hysteria," "basal gangliar disorder (toxic, allergic, heredofamilial, post-infectious, infectious??—or psychiatric?)," as well as amyotrophic lateral sclerosis (Lou Gehrig's disease). He saw a resemblance between kuru and delirium tremens, only the Fore didn't drink. Were metals leaching from their copper-rich streams making them sick? Was kuru a delayed symptom of some earlier infection, or caused by the insects the Fore ate? All these questions remained unanswered— there was no sign of infection, no clear genetic origin, no solid environmental cause, and there were no known previous cases. Kuru seemed "one of the most mystifying and baffling ailments . . . known."

Gajdusek and his band continued to travel from village to village. Not waiting for a diagnosis, he jumped into trying out cures. He treated children with kuru with phenobarbital and cortisone and testosterone, vitamins and antihistamines, low doses of adrenocorticotropic hormone, sulfonamides, chloramphenicol, dimercaprol, and iron supplement. The Fore were a dartboard for his intuitions. Sometimes a sufferer appeared to be improving, but no one got better for long. The graves filled up, but the Fore did not blame Gajdusek, as they had the Australians. Their children trusted him, and that was enough for them. He was thrilled when Fore men—"great pig-tusks through their noses"—smeared him with pig fat as the children flocked around him and chanted "Docta America!" With one hand he shot them full of penicillin while with the other he bled them. Life among these tribespeople could not be better.*

Gajdusek collected more information in a month than the Australians could have managed in a year. Still he made no progress. Melbourne sent back a report on a brain Gajdusek had given them, reporting it showed no significant alterations. The Australians were beginning to believe the disease was genetic. The belief had political implications. With so many Fore women dead, Fore men were beginning to turn to other tribes to find mates. What if they contaminated their neighbors through interbreeding? What if those neighbors in turn went on to marry Europeans or Americans? The Australians proposed a quarantine.

The American labs, meanwhile, were more thorough than their

---

* Bleeding for Gajdusek seems to have been an almost sexual way of making contact with others, especially children. Note, for instance, this journal entry from a July 1956 medical visit to the West Nakansi and Mumusi children of New Britain: "I bled them all without difficulty and as usual, our rapport increased greatly—especially with those urchins I knew less well—after having done the venepunctures!"

Australian counterparts. What they were seeing in their brains was eye-opening—"very spectacular neuronophagia . . . very intense gliosis . . . striking changes affecting Purkinje cells . . . and bizarre deformities of Purkinje-cell dendrites"—all suggestive of severe neurodegenerative disease. Dr. Igor Klatzo, a Russian-born neuropathologist working for the NIH, wrote that the pathology of the disease reminded him of one "described by Jakob and Creutzfeldt" in the 1920s that struck a handful of elderly people leaving holes in their brains. The comparison occurred to him because he had just received a copy of a new handbook of neuropathology. He had been thumbing through it at random when he came upon the entry for the disease. ("Such a luck," he remarks of the coincidence some forty years later.)

But Jakob-Creutzfeldt disease (as it was then called) was just a guess: kuru afflicted a very different population than it—young women and infants. Not surprisingly, then, neither Gajdusek, who had never before heard of Jakob-Creutzfeldt disease, nor any of his overseers seized on the comparison between the two diseases. "Two cases . . . occur in distant, remote hamlets," Gajdusek noted, "in two individuals coming into contact rarely. When the disease strikes the same 'family' or household again, it is living at a different site; often different food-preparers, etc are involved, and it is often years after the death of the first in the family." It was an unsolvable puzzle. Gajdusek bled some more Fore. "The natives evinced some disappointment when we ran out of bleeding-containers," he wrote from Lufa.

Sir Mac had understood that Gajdusek's genius was his energy and his far-flung interests. He was a jack of all trades but not "a first-rate scientist." This limitation was beginning to show. A lot of his work was just makework, as some of his own supporters at the NIH recognized. What was needed, one wrote, was a group of epidemiologists, "with experts in anthropology, genetics, diet and personal habits, and water supply collaborating as a team." Gajdusek wrote back that what they didn't understand was that he *was* that team. He was a one-man (two, if you counted Zigas) army. He pointed out that he was analyzing five hundred foods that the Fore ate. It was a big job, and he had it in hand.

Meanwhile, the press had picked up on kuru. In the brief time that Gajdusek had been among them, the Fore had become tabloid fodder, a "primitive stone-age people" suffering "the laughing death." A *Time* magazine article in 1957 began, "In the eastern highlands of New Guinea, sudden bursts of maniacal laughter shrilled through the walls of many a circular, windowless grass hut, echoing through the surrounding jungle . . ."

The coverage appalled Gajdusek. He felt again his disdain for the West. He decided to take a trip to the Fore's northern border to see the Kukukuku, the fiercest and most difficult of all the tribes, known for the long cassowary feathers they wore as headdresses ("Kukukuku" was a corruption of the tribe's word for cassowary). Gajdusek claimed he was "ready to bleed Kuks galore," but in fact he had become dispirited, wondering whether all this time spent on kuru was worth it. Sir Mac, having discovered that he was also sending brains to the Americans, had terminated contact. The Americans were telling him all this blood-taking was a waste of time. But among the Kukukuku, things turned around. He had found a cache of books at a patrol post, "Joseph Conrad, American verse, Macaulay's speeches, and some Scott Fitzgerald," and devoured them. Better yet, if he was finding no new clues to kuru he found something almost as good, at a Kukukuku hamlet: "In late afternoon," he recorded in his journal, "I wandered again about the village. I was invited into the men's house and here I ate pandanus nuts offered me by the men and boys. In their own village their slight reticence promptly subsided and they were ribald and forward. They insisted on examining me from head to foot, were most insistent upon feeling and observing my genitalia, and made insistent and repeated offers of fellatio, designating a host of willing and ribald youngsters for the role. . . . That all the men and boys are thoroughly familiar and practiced in fellatio is most evident from the readiness with which even pre-pubertal boys make ribald gestures offering their services in fellatio, and from the persistent suggestion to many of our police, to cargo boys, to my mankis [young boys], and to myself that we accept the many willing and insistent fellators. I am most curious to know what role homosexuality plays in their culture." The next day he walked in on some of his cargo boys with Kukukuku boys and wondered whether he had stumbled on "nefarious trade deals" or "a rich orgy of fellatio." Gajdusek was among the "wonderful Kukukukus." He did not find any kuru. But at last he had found the surf.

Carleton Gajdusek left the Kukukuku and Fore region in January 1958, nine months after he got there. He had a post waiting for him under Joseph Smadel at the NIH, but he didn't return to the States immediately. Instead, he traveled in Southeast Asia, returning to the study of children in primitive cultures. In no time he had found new and intriguing problems. "I am having a fascinating time here . . . and already I have spotted a half-dozen new problems—some good!!" he teased Smadel, but in fact he was always thinking about kuru and when he got back to the NIH in late 1958 he turned his attention to it.

There remained two main theories of what caused the disease. The more accepted one was that the Fore suffered from a genetic defect. The problem was how could a mutation as lethal and widespread as kuru exist? Evolutionary theory required that such a mutation would also have to confer some enormous offsetting advantage on the population that contained it, and it was hard to imagine what advantage could compensate for widespread early death.

Infection was the second theory—and it had been the earliest. Infection had been on Gajdusek's mind when he and Zigas first teamed up, driving their van with two kuru patients (in Zigas's words: "my overseas guest, the two belles doomed to join their ancestors and I") from Kainantu to Okapa in March 1957. But the evidence against infection was hard to get around: if kuru was an infection, why didn't it track as one? Infections caused fevers and provoked antibodies that left telltale traces in the blood and the spinal fluid. Kuru did none of these things. Gajdusek's best explanation was that a protozoan, a fungus, or a *Toxoplasma* parasite might be involved because all could cause disease almost without an immune system response. The problem was that the epidemiological information gave no evidence such agents had infected the Fore.

Remarkable as he was, Gajdusek could not crack kuru on his own. His detractors at the NIH had a point: what was needed was a team of anthropologists and epidemiologists—people with different personalities, prejudices, and skills.

In the end, it was two anthropologists who solved the kuru mystery. A husband and wife team from Australia, Robert and Shirley Glasse, came to the Fore in the 1960s, sent by the Australian government to draw up a pedigree of all the victims of kuru and show how the sick were related to one another. The Fore did not share the Western idea of family; they did not make a clear distinction between friends and relations, and unraveling this complexity to draw valid genealogies was going to take someone trained in data collection a lot of work. The Australians thought that was fine: anthropologists were cheaper than doctors and would put up with worse living conditions.

The Glasses set up camp in a Fore village and, unlike Gajdusek, they stayed put. They spent their time in conversation with the Fore, afternoon "talk-talks," carefully tracing who had lived with whom in what hamlet when. Shirley Glasse was able to get women, the primary victims of kuru, to open up to her. Gajdusek's research was always scattershot: a number of colleagues recalled that he did not speak the local languages as well as he thought he did and he was not always sure where he was or who he was talking to. He was always really more interested in his own words than anyone else's. One patrol officer remembered a Gajdusek visit this way: "this strange white bloke would appear out of the bush, jabber at you in a language you didn't understand, stick a needle into you, write something in a book, and then move on." Gajdusek departed with so many blood samples it took teams of porters to carry them out.

In addition, Gajdusek's medical literacy also turned out to be a disadvantage in the case of kuru. The Glasses had no scientific preconceptions to pen up their thoughts. They were open to ideas that Gajdusek wasn't. They teased out a fascinating story of culture, change—and cannibalism.

One of the salient facts surrounding kuru was that the Fore said it was of recent origin. If you believed that, then whatever was causing the disease in their midst must be new too, and much was lately new for the Fore. When their Highlands neighbors showed them sweet potato, they replaced taro with it in their diet. When their neighbors showed them how to tame wild pigs, they adopted the practice, too. The patrol officers pressed chicken on them. Suddenly the Fore were in the chicken business.

As the Glasses learned, the custom of eating human flesh had also come to the Fore from the outside, about fifty years before. The belief that the Fore were cannibals was widespread among locals and Westerners, the villagers "cheerfully admit[ing] to cannibal practices," as a patrol report by R. I. Skinner on the Fore noted in 1947. What wasn't known was that cannibalism was new to them. The Northern Fore had picked up cannibalism from the Kamano to the north, whose greater sophistication was legendary among the tribes. The Southern Fore admired the Northern Fore and acquired the habit in turn from them. As one Fore described the process, "It so happened that an ancestor . . . named Tawazi was killed by . . . sorcery. After his death the body was carried to Krawanti where it was cooked and portions of the meat distributed throughout the district. People tasting it expressed their approval. 'This is sweet,' they said, 'What is the matter with us, are we mad? Here is good food and we have neglected to eat it.' " Game in the forests was giving out due to the increasing population, and, though no one was starving, the Fore knew a good idea when they saw it. "The thing you have to remember about the Fore's cannibalism is they thought human flesh was delicious. They enjoyed it," Shirley Glasse (now Lindenbaum) says.

Many tribes were said to eat their enemies as an act of vengeance, and this practice had entered European mythology, but revenge cannibalism was not the Fore's practice. They loved their dead and mourned them first, but after mourning, they got down to culinary business. The Fore were expert butchers, able with stone tools to make cuts a pathologist would admire.

The meal was symbolic as well as nutritious. The Fore experienced burial as a kind of digestion: the ground ate the body and was enriched by it. That humans could be food was consistent with their worldview, which was essentially oral. "I eat you," was a common greeting, much to the surprise of early patrol officers and anthropologists. Play biting was a part of growing up, and the Fore used body parts as metaphors for relationships of importance: your best friend was your "umbilical cord," your wife, your "hand." You ate your dead, then, also to reconnect with them. (The Fore never ate their own children or grandchildren, though: that they saw as incest, which was taboo.)

In Fore communities, pigs were used to link individuals to one another through reciprocal obligation—I eat your pig. You eat mine. We are friends. The goal was strategic, in a society where war between friends was permanent. Something similar was intended with the consumption of human bodies. The different parts of the body were given out according to a code of obligation and payment. For instance, if the deceased was female, her daughters-in-law got the arms and legs, her sisters-in-law the buttocks, intestine, and vulva. If the deceased was male, the testicles went to his uncles' wives. The ceremonial exchanges served to bind different village groups in a union of mutual obligation that helped limit the violent skirmishes among hamlets. Any person who was invited to sit down and given food left both honored and well fed, improving the prospects for alliances with his host, at least for the moment.

The Glasses did not have medical degrees; they could not explicitly identify the cause of kuru. But they had drawn a road map for anyone who cared to follow it: the Fore had begun eating human flesh at around the time kuru had begun showing up among them. The Glasses' work was substantiated by a young Australian doctor named John Mathews, who contributed a careful epidemiological correlation of Fore funeral feasts and outbreaks of kuru. Gajdusek resisted their conclusion, partially because he hated to be scooped.

But the shifts in the pattern of kuru infection over time left no doubt that the Glasses and Mathews were right. The missionaries who came with the Australians in the fifties opposed cannibalism. The Fore, always agreeable, abandoned it. By the early to mid-1960s it was probably gone. Around that time, children stopped dying of the disease. Then young people did. Finally, only elderly women were affected. Here were great clues for the epidemiologists. The Fore were no longer doing something they had previously done that had made them ill, and it had to be something women and children had done much more often than men. Paradoxically, Gajdusek had been closest to a solution before he had started his investigations. In his first diary entry on the disease, fresh from outmaneuvering Anderson and Sir Mac but before he'd seen a sufferer, he wrote, "The South Fore adults and children have until recently been eating their dead relatives in a ceremonial cannibalism. . . . Women and children, particularly, partake of the human flesh." A week later he wrote Smadel that a kuru victim's body had just been fed to some children. A culture that fed diseased corpses to women and children? The clues had been there and he had briefly considered them. What he could not get past was that kuru did not look like an infection, so any speculation about how the infection occurred seemed pointless. He did try to get around this problem: he floated the idea that the Fore were first exposed to human flesh as young children and then developed an allergy to it, so that when they sampled it later in life it was lethal to them—along the model, say, of bee stings.

There were two problems with this scenario. In Gajdusek's day, cannibalism no longer appeared widespread enough to account for the thousands of kuru deaths; no one was thinking in terms of a disease that lay dormant for decades, the way prion diseases would turn out to. A bigger objection was that autoimmune reactions, like infections, leave their footprints in the blood, and the blood of the kuru victims had no such traces. As a result, Gajdusek's kuru investigations had come to naught, one of the great near-misses of modern epidemiology.

Gajdusek wanted to solve two mysteries, though: not just what caused kuru but how, and his contribution would come with the latter when he identified the mechanism of the disease and aspects of the novel nature of the organism behind it. Thanks to his energy, everyone in the scientific world heard about "slow viruses," as he took to calling the agent behind kuru and such related diseases as Creutzfeldt-Jakob disease and scrapie, and scientists threw resources at slow viruses until they began to yield their secrets. His work would change our understanding of disease.

Of course, from the Fore point of view, neither the Glasses nor Gajdusek nor the millions of dollars spent bleeding and later genotyping them over the past four decades has made any difference. No one has ever survived kuru. The death toll is by now around three thousand. Cannibalism has been absent from New Guinea for forty years, yet a few old Fore women still die every year of the disease. So in the end it was neither Gajdusek nor the Glasses but Apekono who was right when—at least, in Vincent Zigas's imaginative recounting—he ordered the doctor to put away his Sloane's Liniment fifty years ago. Western medicine was no match for the Fore's "strong sorcery."

CHAPTER 6

MONKEY BUSINESS BETHESDA, MARYLAND, *1965*

It has even been suggested that kuru be described
as the "disease of theories."

— JOHN MATHEWS, M.D. thesis,
University of Melbourne, 1971

At the NIH, Carleton Gajdusek wanted to focus on what caused kuru and Joe Smadel was willing to give him the resources to figure it out. Smadel took Gajdusek's program on "Child Growth and Development and Disease Patterns in Primitive Cultures" and folded it into the Division of Collaborative and Field Research in the National Institute of Neurological Diseases and Blindness. Although he remained thoroughly unconventional (he didn't own a suit until a Swedish friend bought one for him for the Nobel Prize ceremony almost twenty years later), Gajdusek found a place in the Western establishment he had tried so hard to escape.

In theory, Gajdusek reported to Smadel, but in practice he could do what he wanted, how he wanted. Gajdusek came home believing kuru was hereditary (the Glasses had not yet done their field research) but he was not committed to the idea. In 1959, he got some information that made him reexamine the possibility of infection. In 1947, the first modern American case of scrapie appeared, in a flock of sheep in Michigan. The U.S. Department of Agriculture began sending veterinarians to England to learn about the disease with which the English had so much experience. In 1959, one of the American investigators, a veterinarian pathologist named William Hadlow, happened to see an exhibit on kuru at the Wellcome Medical Museum in London. It included photomicrographs of kuru brain tissue by Igor Klatzo and Gajdusek's photographs of the disease's victims. Until he saw the kuru exhibit, Hadlow remembered, he had never seen a disease that left holes in the brain the way scrapie did. He felt as if he were seeing the same slides he had sitting back in his lab. He was excited enough to write a note to *Lancet,* the British medical journal, noting an "overall resemblance" between scrapie and kuru that was "uncanny" and urging research to bring the connection to light. He also sent a copy of his letter directly to "the one person who would be interested in it": Gajdusek.

Hadlow was not really telling Gajdusek anything more than Klatzo had when he had compared kuru to Jakob-Creutzfeldt disease: Your disease with no known cause resembles my disease with no known cause. The difference was that while virtually nothing was known about Jakob-Creutzfeldt disease—it was still "a convenient dumping ground for otherwise unclassifiable dementias"—a significant body of information had grown up around scrapie in the previous century. The disease had never disappeared since the great outbreak of the late 1700s—it remained at low levels with periodic surges. Each wave prompted new research on the disease, research that dried up when the wave retreated. But the mysterious disease was slowly being understood. In the 1930s, two French veterinarians injected healthy sheep with tissue from scrapie-affected sheep. They had been trying to figure out whether scrapie was infectious or inherited, an inquiry that ended inconclusively many times before. This time, because they had noticed that sheep on farms rarely got scrapie before they were two years old, they gave the disease time to manifest itself. After fourteen months, one sheep got sick, and after twenty-two months, a second one did.

Meanwhile, in Scotland, an accidental experiment brought the same conclusion. In 1935, English researchers led by a veterinarian named W. S. Gordon conducted a trial with a vaccine they had manufactured for louping-ill. Louping-ill is a tick-borne virus that causes sheep to hop or leap as they walk. The size of Gordon's louping-ill vaccine trial was enormous: forty thousand sheep. He had prepared his inoculant by taking tissue from infected sheep's brains, mashing it up, and removing the infectivity with a chemical—in this case formalin, a diluted version of formaldehyde. Nothing survives formaldehyde. This is ideal in a vaccine, because a dead virus is exactly what the researcher wants. It won't make the animal sick, but the dead viruses will still provoke an immune response. The antibodies from that immune response will remain in the blood and keep the animal from getting sick if it is exposed to a live virus later on.

Gordon's experiment worked, in that his sheep developed immunity to louping-ill. But two years later, hundreds of them began coming down with scrapie. About fifteen hundred sheep got sick in all, according to Gordon's report, though this estimate is probably too low, because many of the sheep were sold off or butchered before scrapie began to make its appearance. Gordon realized that he had been using sheep brain that contained not just dead louping-ill virus, but also whatever the agent was that caused scrapie. By injecting it, he had spread the scrapie to the flock. The veterinarian repeated the experiment to confirm his suspicion and thousands more sheep died.

It was now clear that sheep could catch scrapie—at least from a needle—and that the disease's symptoms made their appearance very slowly. The information provided an essential clue to the mystery of kuru as well. Before leaving the Highlands, Gajdusek had come across a kuru victim who had died on the Papuan coast, years after leaving the Fore region. He asked Smadel how the NIH toxicologists could explain an infection that remained asymptomatic for months, even years. W. S. Gordon's botched louping-ill experiment seemed to provide an answer.

Gajdusek, who had never before heard of scrapie, did not respond to Hadlow's letter with candor: he told the scrapie researcher he already had transmission experiments underway to transmit kuru to animals, when in fact he had only made a few efforts in that direction while still trying to figure out a genetic explanation for the disease. Struck by Hadlow's idea, he now threw himself into trying to prove kuru was infectious. He stocked up on everything from mice to hamsters to chimpanzees and started injecting them with kuru homogenate. In 1961, he and Joe Smadel offered Hadlow the job of overseeing the experiments. Hadlow declined, saying he did not want to be an "exalted handler of apes."

Primates were central to Gajdusek's program: overall, he says, he ran through about a thousand chimpanzees (a figure that surely is exaggerated). Chimps were the gold standard if you were interested in human disease, because they were humans' closest relatives. But chimps had drawbacks. "You didn't want to keep a chimp if you could possibly avoid it," remembered Paul Brown, a researcher who worked with Gajdusek at his NIH lab. "They were incredibly expensive. Incredibly strong. And they lived a long time." They also had a way of making the researchers quite upset. "We were all very attached to them," Michael Alpers, the head of the kuru research program in Okapa, remembered. The lab secretary would take the chimps home every night in her car and drive them to work the next day. One researcher kept a baby chimp as a pet.

The job of running the animal infection experiments ultimately went to C. J. Gibbs, a virus researcher whom Gajdusek had met when, as an Army captain at Walter Reed, he had given the new recruit an inoculation. Gibbs complemented Gajdusek well: he was accessible, empathetic, and practical, and he did not care about credit. Gibbs obtained the chimps from what Alpers remembers as "dodgy dealers in Florida," and was able to get authorization from the federal agency that was the precursor to the U.S. Fish and Wildlife Service to open up a small monkey house on a five-thousand-acre wildlife preserve at the Patuxent Wildlife Research Center. Bio-security was nonexistent: on a visit in the mid-1960s, William Hadlow remembered walking out to see the chimps and having them spit in his face. Gajdusek began his experiments on "6 chimpanzees, 32 rhesus monkeys, 25 cynomolgi [macaques] and 10 African green monkeys" in 1962 and 1963, and promised not to give up "before five years." The technique by which scientists tested an agent for infectivity—inject, wait, autopsy—was essentially unchanged since Pasteur's time. Once he had the transmission experiments under way, Gajdusek took off again for foreign places; if kuru was like scrapie, nothing was going to happen anytime soon.

The arrangement was very congenial to him. He thought he could do better thinking in primitive places. Plus, he had left behind a hospital in Okapa, and the Fore expected him to return. In Okapa he could add to his supply of kuru brains, the fresher the better. Gajdusek even sent Paul Brown with liquid hydrogen to Okapa to freeze brains as soon as they came out of the victims' skulls, so as to preserve the best possible chance that the infectious agent in them didn't die before the researchers at Patuxent could inject it into the chimps. Meanwhile, Gajdusek went wherever the winds took him—New Guinea and elsewhere—often touching down among the Anga or other tribes with pedophiliac traditions. He even adopted a twelve-year-old Anga boy, who arrived at Dulles Airport in 1963 in bare feet and with a bone through his nose.

—

Georgette, one of the chimps at Patuxent, began to grow sick in June 1965, twenty-one months after she had been injected with kuru. As usual, Gajdusek was traveling. The lab called him back from New Guinea. "He came rather grudgingly," Alpers remembered, expecting "a false alarm: But the chimp performed magnificently, dragging herself around, shaking, looking for all the world like a kuru patient." The lab ran the same blood tests they had run in New Guinea on kuru victims, looking for dietary contaminants or metal poisoning; the lead in the bars on their cage was a candidate. The tests were negative. Another chimp, Daisy, became ill. As each chimp got sicker, he or she was given a mattress and twenty-four-hour nursing care, while Gajdusek ushered in what Gibbs calls "a plethora of nationally and internationally recognized neurologists" to see them. Then Gajdusek hit the road, barnstorming around various research facilities with his news, beginning the task of knitting kuru into some broader disease idea. Alan Dickinson, a scrapie researcher at the Moredun Institute in Scotland, remembered "Gajd showing up with a film reel of kuru and his toothbrush." The animals became weaker and weaker, able only to slide across their cages to get their food with their mouths on the ground. Like the human victims of kuru—and much as Pietro knew the name Tosca—the chimps kept their higher cortical function, the knowledge of who and where they were, to the end. An animal "in the terminal phase would still turn her head at the whisper of her name," Alpers remembered.

Gajdusek arranged for a British pathologist who had seen a lot of scrapie to fly in after the chimps died and examine their brains. She saw enough similarity to draw a parallel to what she had seen in kuru victims whose tissue she had examined. The chimps had died of what killed the Fore. It was a moment of triumph for Gajdusek and his lab. Here was proof kuru was not a genetic disease but an infectious one.

—

Gajdusek remained intrigued by Igor Klatzo's comparison of kuru to Creutzfeldt-Jakob disease, as the disease was now called.* So the lab began inoculating healthy chimps with tissue from sufferers of the mysterious neuromuscular disease next. After around a year, these chimps also grew sick. When the animals died, pathologists examined their brains and saw that the sponginess and the holes resembled those of the kuru-infected chimps and other chimps who had been inoculated with scrapie. One, as the saying goes, was a novelty; two was a coincidence; three—kuru, CJD, and scrapie—was a theory. Gajdusek published the results of his tests in 1968 and 1969. These long-ignored diseases, he declared, were caused by the same thing: some sort of novel, hard to destroy, slow-acting virus. His idea, he knew, was vague. He was not really sure what he meant by it and neither was anyone else.

The key sticking point was the word "virus." Viruses are essentially bits of nucleic acid covered by protein; they insert themselves into cells and trick the cell's reproductive apparatus into copying them. A virus can make thousands of copies of itself in a day. As foreign objects in the cell, viruses generally provoke an immune reaction in their unwilling host, and it is these antibodies that usually reveal the strain of the virus. Though they are not technically alive, viruses do contain bits of DNA (or RNA), so they can be neutralized by the same techniques that kill living things—everything from washing with soap and water, to heating, to irradiation. And most viruses, once they are removed from the cell that they are parasitizing, die on their own, usually in a few hours.

Gajdusek's "odd, slow viruses" had none of these attributes, as he knew. For instance, you could get ordinary viruses to grow in petri

---

* C. J. Gibbs says he rearranged "Jakob-Creutzfeldt disease" so the initials would match his own, but Gajdusek claims the change was his doing: "I thought Creutzfeldt had done better work."

dishes full of cells, but the scrapie agent, whatever its nature, did not grow outside its host. The only way to study it was to inject scrapie-infected tissue into live animals and wait for them to get sick. The average virus experiment took about a week; the average scrapie experiment took two years.

This made scrapie research frustrating work. (One British committee recommended that researchers in the field be chosen "with as much care as are astronauts.") The ideal researcher had great perseverance—and was often quite eccentric. Quintessential was D. R. Wilson at the Moredun Institute in Scotland, who worked in the middle of the last century for more than a decade trying, with mounting frustration, to kill the scrapie agent. He found that it survived desiccation; dosing with chloroform, phenol, and formalin; ultraviolet light; and cooking at 100 degrees centigrade for thirty minutes. The scrapie researcher Alan Dickinson told me he remembered Wilson at the end of his career as "very, very, very quiet. Of course, that was after his breakdown." In the end, Wilson published only one paper, recounting his attempts to destroy the strange virus.

But slowly researchers, especially in Britain, began to establish certain attributes of the scrapie virus. The South African–born radiologist Tikvah Alper was an independent-minded and committed researcher who in her spare time helped her husband, a famous anthrax researcher, develop an improved technique for bacteria analysis.* In the mid-1960s, she grew intrigued by the unique properties of the scrapie agent and tried irradiating it with a mercury heat lamp at her London lab. She found that radiation, which kills all living things, did not kill

* Alper refused a Royal sixtieth wedding anniversary greeting from the queen because the queen issued it to her and her husband under his last name. Buckingham Palace relented and the greeting went out to Dr. Max Sterne and Dr. Tikvah Alper. "I suppose the other way around would have been too much to hope for," Alper commented.

the scrapie particle. At roughly the same time, Alan Dickinson of the Moredun Institute and others found that there were different strains of scrapie, identifiable by the pattern of damage they left in the sheep's body. These facts added up to a very strange infectious principle indeed: a particle that had strains like a virus but didn't die under conditions that would kill a virus and that the body didn't recognize as foreign. Gajdusek, who was following these discoveries, refined his thinking. He now theorized that the infectious agent might be "a well-known virus . . . modified into a defective, incomplete, or highly integrated or repressed agent in vivo." In other words, scrapie might be a bit of outside DNA or RNA so small or so oddly shaped or so cleverly disguised in the body's native proteins that it sneaked in under the body's immune system radar.

Other researchers went further, proposing that the scrapie virus was no virus at all. Viruses are made up of a core of malignant nucleic acid covered by protein. (The geneticist Peter Medawar once described them as "bad news wrapped in a protein coat.") The odd thing about scrapie was that everyone could find the coat—when you spun the scrapie particle at high speeds in a centrifuge, plenty of bits of protein detached—but no one could find the DNA. Was it because there wasn't any in the infectious agent? Could an infectious agent be entirely made of protein?

The conventional wisdom was no. Proteins are accumulations of ordinary molecules. They are the building blocks and engines and messengers of the body—about 50 percent of the nonwater weight of a cell comes from its proteins—but they themselves are not alive. Because they are not living, proteins maintain their function in a lot of environments that destroy life. For instance, proteins can be exposed to detergents and radiation and some will still function. Formalin won't reliably destroy them. But to suggest, as some researchers began to in the late 1960s, that a protein could make copies of itself in the victim's body—that a nonliving agent was somehow replicating itself or being replicated in the victim's body without any DNA and causing disease—pushed up against the impossible. Proteins were just physical structures, not proactive ones. They were no more alive, and no more infectious, than bone.

So most researchers who considered the scrapie problem continued to believe that a tiny virus was hiding alongside or within the scrapie protein. The few who dissented were not taken very seriously. One was Tikvah Alper. Another was the British scrapie researcher I. H. Pattison, who showed in the 1960s that the scrapie agent behaved a lot like the allergic encephalitis agent, a protein that triggered an autoimmune disorder. "My own non-viral suggestion of a small protein was dismissed as buffoonery," he wrote in a 1992 remembrance. A professor of veterinary medicine named Tony Palmer, who kept a flock of scrapie-infected sheep on the roof of Queen's Hospital in London, suggested "a non-protein moiety, perhaps carbohydrate which on introduction into the body forms a template for the subsequent reduplication of the agent." He had, in fact, stumbled on the key behind the replication of infectious proteins. But he put the suggestion in the last sentence of his essay in a 1960 book called *Progress in the Biological Sciences in Relation to Dermatology,* where no one saw it.

The most memorable attempt to establish the possibility of a self-replicating protein came from a mathematician at Bedford College in London, J. S. Griffith. Griffith had figured briefly in James Watson's and Francis Crick's discovery of the structure of DNA as a colleague who believed conventional chemical reactions were the key to understanding gene replication. Watson thought his insistence was a little backward: DNA was the thing to look at. Fourteen years later, Griffith was still interested in proving that chemistry could explain biological processes, and this time he got it right. He would become the founding theorist in the prion field.

In 1967, he posited three ways a protein could replicate itself. Two of his ideas were little more than parlor games. One asked, What if there was a gene that made a protein whose function was to switch on the gene that made it? If so, then infecting the gene with that protein would be tantamount to reproducing the protein. Another idea was that a foreign body in a host happened to be the same as the antibody produced by that host in response to the invasion. Then the invading antigen would cause the body to make more of itself. Though this was a clever hypothesis, there was no example of such a mechanism in nature; Griffith himself dismissed the idea, because he knew that no one had ever found either antigen or antibodies where scrapie was concerned.

Griffith's last idea—the one that clicked in researchers' minds—was that proteins could convert other proteins from one form to another using a positive feedback mechanism, a kind of forward catalyst, as happened in chemical reactions. For example, if you dissolve salt in boiling water and then put it in a jar and cover it and put it in the refrigerator with a string hanging down from the lid, the salt will crystallize as it cools, starting with the molecules along the string. On a molecular level, subatomic forces are causing each molecule to align itself with the molecules that have already lined themselves up. The string acts as the seed, the equivalent of the first deformed protein. "With such a mechanism," Griffith wrote, "it would be easy to understand the spontaneous appearance of the disease in previously unaffected animals." All you needed was one misshapen molecule to start things off. One of the appealing things about nucleation, as this feed-forward loop is called, was that it allowed for a kind of replication that had nothing to do with DNA.

This represented a surprising return to an idea put forward in the nineteenth century by the chemist Baron Justus von Liebig and his friend Friedrich Wöhler, the synthesizer of urea. In opposition to Louis Pasteur, they had argued that there was nothing unique about disease, any more than there was about life in general. Instead, both were just the product of molecules behaving according to the laws of chemical bonds. Griffith's idea would explain why you could stop scrapie only by denaturing the scrapie protein. It would also explain why there were no antibodies to the protein in sufferers from FFI, like Pietro and his family, or from sufferers of Creutzfeldt-Jakob disease; the lethal proteins came from the victims themselves.

Griffith was not well placed to confute biology's central dogma—he was a mathematician who dabbled in neuroscience. His third idea smacked of not-very-well-informed extrapolation. But, over time, it would be consistently cited by researchers finding their way to a solution to the scrapie and CJD mystery.

Gajdusek watched the back-and-forth over proteins and DNA. He was not ready to commit his prestige to the protein-only point of view. While he gingerly associated himself with the possibility that there was no DNA in the kuru or scrapie agent, at the same time he never cut his ties to the people who believed there was. Meanwhile, he kept the field in public view as no one else could, helped by a personal mailing list of more than a thousand interested scientists.

In 1976, the Karolinska Institute awarded him the Nobel Prize in physiology or medicine for discovering "a completely new type of infectious agent." Friends, on hearing the news, wondered whether it was for medicine or literature. Certainly, the Institute was rewarding him for doing the key experiments in the field (showing the agent was transmissible) and for the expert framing of a question (was infection possible without a living agent?) rather than for answering it. No one knew, yet, whether a virus or something odder caused kuru or, for that matter, CJD and scrapie, but there was clearly a group of diseases out there that were not like conventional ones. Gajdusek had a theory of how these diseases were connected. It went like this: the scrapie agent began as a disease of sheep and passed, through "kitchen and butchery accidents involving the contamination of skin and eyes," into humans, where it manifested itself as CJD. One person infected with CJD by chance died in New Guinea and the Fore ate him; the disease then showed up in his unlucky diners as kuru. In his Nobel acceptance speech, Gajdusek said that though scrapie and kuru were "infectious particles unique in the biology of replicating infectious agents . . . these viruses still demonstrate sufficiently classical behavior of other infectious microbial agents for us to retain, perhaps with misgivings, the title of 'viruses.' " He went on: "A major effort in my laboratory has been and is now being directed toward the molecular biological elucidation of the nature and structure of this group of atypical viruses." That effort would prove, he said, that all the transmissible viral spongiform encephalopathies—scrapie, kuru, and Creutzfeldt-Jakob disease—were really one.

CHAPTER 7

"BOH!" THE VENETO, *1973*

What on earth did this woman die of?
     —A PATHOLOGIST IN PADUA
      examining Assunta

t was 1973. The Veneto was in the middle of a typically hot summer. When the summer heat comes, it not only wafts in from the lagoon but bubbles out of the irrigation ditches and seems to ooze up from the wet fields. The *patrizi* are long gone, their villas owned by young professionals. The Italians eliminated malarial mosquitoes in the 1960s with helicopters and DDT, but still, in the Venetan mind it remains an unhealthy heat and anyone who can get away from it does.

After the Second World War, the center of the Veneto moved from Venice to Mestre, its squat, ugly sister city across the lagoon. Venice was old; Mestre was new. Venice had canals; Mestre had streets. Venice had museums; Mestre had stores. The things of the new Italy poured into the streets of Mestre: cars, kitchen sinks, shiny ceramic tiles. For Italians, it was pleasant to leave the past behind.

Almost thirty years after Pietro's death from the family disease, his daughter Assunta was living in a new four-story apartment building in Mestre with her brother, Silvano. She was forty-eight, had never married, and had long been a wool knitter. For years she'd worked from her home, and then had taken a job at a small factory to knit sweaters for other companies.

Her nimble hands could fashion things that the world wanted, things that companies like Stefanel and Benetton could sell and that could finally give the Veneto an economic life outside of farming and that also left women like Assunta time to do the hidden work they were expected to do—the cooking, washing, ironing, and sewing, while men spent their evenings out. Assunta was not one of those women in black skirts with head scarves who scowl at foreigners. She wore attractive clothes, summer or winter—skirts and blouses and sometimes knitted tops. Her hair was short and sometimes she highlighted it with henna. But despite her modern trappings, she was religious, still the teenager praying for her father's recovery, a modest and fearful woman.

Stepping down from a bus one day on a visit to Chioggia, an old fishing town at the southern end of the lagoon, Assunta felt a shock. It began at the top of her head and then went all the way down to her feet—a sizzling in her entire nervous system. The sensation was so powerful that she grabbed onto the side of the bus. Then came a moment of intense dizziness. Then the vertigo passed.

Was it the heat? Had she not eaten? Could it be something more serious? The papers were reporting outbreaks of cholera along the Adriatic, the old Venice nipping at the new.

In the days that followed, she had another, smaller shock. She felt listless. She felt hot. But then again, it was August. You could not expect to feel well in the summer heat. Any Italian knew that to stay in town was the height of folly. During the summer months, she sometimes went with Silvano and her mother to Jesolo, where her father,

Pietro, had planned to build a hotel before he fell ill. Others had built a summer resort there for the growing Venetan middle class—a beach-front town with restaurants and outdoor bands and low stucco condos in happy colors like coral and chartreuse, not a spot of nature as far as the eye could see. Silvano came and went to Jesolo in his BMW on weekends, taking his mother and sister out dancing in the evenings. The apartment was Silvano's—he was a generous, loving brother who gracefully supported the family.

There were tens of thousands of Venetans at Jesolo that summer. They danced and walked down the pedestrian malls and gossiped about the shortages due to OPEC's recent embargo on oil. In America, it caused inconvenience, but in Italy the embargo struck with enormous force. There were shortages of gas and electricity, and in response the government announced a period of *semi-austerità.*

Being hampered in their desires was not pleasant to Italians. The old class bitterness that had so often divided Italy quickly came out anew. The unions—the ENCL, the SEAI—threatened strikes. The bus drivers went on a slowdown. Food was short on the shelves and there was a government telephone number to call to report price gouging, but it was always busy.

Over the next two weeks, Assunta did not feel better. She told her family she was at the very limit of exhaustion. Her eyes looked glazed, and she held her head stiffly. She had always been a little anxious, but now she was more so. She felt like a marionette whose master had dropped the strings. She was always tired. Even if she slept, she didn't wake up refreshed. What was upsetting her? She had recently ended a friendship with a married man and just now she stopped menstruating. She had never had any children and, suddenly, she never would. She'd helped to raise Silvano and her niece Lisi. One year she'd worked at a summer daycare program, taking children to museums and the beach. Italy was full of children. How she loved them!

Silvano knew what was happening and so did their mother, but they had each seen a half-dozen relatives die of the family disease and had trained themselves not to notice. Assunta was not herself, they would say: that was it, she was tired, perhaps depressed. Her eyes were dark and small. Lisi asked Assunta what was wrong and she told her that she was allergic to light. "I'm so tired," she said. The family decided to find help. Assunta could hardly go to a hospital. What symptoms did she have? Menopause? Nerves? Insomnia? So the family selected a rest home instead, a *casa di cura*. A *casa di cura* was something like a small hospital. Most important, it was private. In a *casa di cura,* doctors could do the necessary tests. The family could come and go as they pleased. Assunta would be protected from some of the stress that seemed to be weighing on her, and her dignity would be preserved. A modest woman, she was not in the habit of being poked and prodded.

The family checked Assunta in on August 20. The doctors too junior to be on vacation took blood samples and a personal history. Assunta told them about her menopause, her difficulty in sleeping, and the shock she felt when she'd gotten off the bus. Observing her over two weeks, they found her problem: she had Meniere's disease. That made sense. Meniere's disease, a disorder of the inner ear, made you feel dizzy and sweat. You became disoriented. The cause of Meniere's disease was unknown; it might be an autoimmune disease or a viral one. Some doctors thought it was connected to menopause. Usually, it went away on its own. It was the perfect diagnosis in August for a rest home in a country of shortages.

Lisi and Ignazio, her boyfriend, a medical school student, came to visit Assunta at the *casa di cura* and saw how quickly she was deteriorating. Watching her unsteady gait as she walked down the corridor, they knew her problem could not be Meniere's disease, but they did not know what it could be. Assunta talked about how noise had begun to bother her. At night she tried to sleep. In a way she did sleep: her eyes closed. She was still. Time passed. Yet when she woke up, she never felt rested. Her forehead was bathed in sweat.

After two weeks, a diagnosis made, Assunta was sent home. It was September. Other Italians were in the midst of the *rientrata,* the return to work. Street lights were out. *Il Gazzettino* showed pictures of empty shelves on the front page. All the same, Italians got by, as they always did, bartering or borrowing what they needed through cousins and friends of cousins. Assunta had started a new job in the spring as a custodian of a school, the sort of state-guaranteed job that an ailing woman could do. The school was in Chioggia and she expected to return to it, but the first few times she took the bus to work, the ride exhausted her. She did not look well, either. There were dark circles around her eyes and her mouth was now stiff on the side, as if the marionette master had picked up a single string and was pulling it.

Assunta thought about going to the mountains, to Recoaro, about forty miles away in the foothills of the Alps, where the air was cooler. Recoaro was a spa town. At the end of the Venetian Republic its waters and treatments were so central to the well-being of the Venetian kidney, liver, and intestines that the Serenissima declared it a public trust. Italians still believed in spa treatments at least somewhat—not as much as they believed in antibiotics, say, but more than in the *massariól.* In Recoaro, there would be fresh air and pretty views. She had never liked the heat and she was always hot these days. In Recoaro, she could continue to improve, and then she would go back to work.

But she never got to Recoaro. Each night in Mestre, she would get a little fever, a *febbricola.* She felt another shock, too, as if she'd stuck her finger in an electric outlet. The sleeplessness worsened. Assunta would lie down but nothing would happen. She would stare at the ceiling, perfectly aware of where she was and how far away sleep felt. Often she thought of babies.

A few weeks later, Assunta went one day to see her mother in the house in which Pietro had died and in which her mother and her sister Isolina were now living. With the rest of the Veneto, the family's ancestral town had grown richer and less provincial. In 1966, the town priest had turned around to face the congregants during mass; three years later, he began reciting the sacred words in Italian instead of Latin. *Dio, non sono degno.* God, I am not worthy. And, in 1971, when vandals snuck into the church tower at night and rang the newly electrified church bells over and over—ordinarily an indication that a flood was on the way or that the pope had died—most townspeople just stayed in bed or kept watching TV.

After her arrival, Assunta went upstairs to try to take a nap. Lisi was also visiting. Isolina gestured for her daughter to follow her and showed Lisi her aunt on the second floor, asleep in the same room in which Pietro had died, mumbling, thrashing her legs, and rubbing the sheets together in her hands. Her mother said to Lisi, "See, that. That's exactly what your grandfather did."

Lisi was shocked. "But I thought you said Grandpa died of encephalitis?"

Her mother shook her head slowly. They went downstairs where her grandmother, seeing their faces, told Lisi simply that there was nothing to be done and that Assunta would die the same way her husband had but would say nothing more. Lisi went back up and woke Assunta. Her aunt smiled at her and said, "Oh, I was dreaming of you as a baby. I was swaddling you. Why am I still so tired?"

By this time it was obvious to everyone that the diagnosis of Meniere's disease was wrong. It could explain the sweating and the dizziness, but not the speed with which Assunta was failing nor her restless dreams. Assunta hadn't had a good night's sleep in weeks. She cried constantly. The family took her to a hospital in Dolo, twenty miles down the new highway from Mestre, where there was a good neurology department. The first thing the doctors there did was treat her insomnia, with Valium. But instead of helping her to sleep, Valium struck a spark in her brain. She fell into an agitated trance. She had terrible nightmares—vast, unending conturbations that left her shaking in her bed and crying. Her legs thrashed, her hands worked constantly. Once the Valium wore off, she was worse than before: she kept getting thinner no matter how much she ate; her sweating got worse, and so did her tremors. The neurologists diagnosed cervical arthrosis and treated her with heat lamps to reduce the swelling, without success. Three weeks after Assunta checked in, she was discharged with a diagnosis of psychoneurotic depression and anxiety. Back home she was affectless, depressed, crying all the time. At night she dreamed of babies. Or, suddenly, she would get up, still asleep, and say she had to leave, frightening whoever was watching over her in her bed.

Italians didn't abandon family members when they got sick. They brought them home. The home was still the place where a person got the best care. But by December the family was exhausted. Casting around for a solution, they decided to take Assunta to the hospital in Padua. Padua was twice as far from Mestre as Dolo. For Assunta, it was like going to another country.

In reborn Italy, after a century and a half of eclipse, Padua had recaptured much of its prestige—at the least, it was home to the best medical school in the country. Padovans still remembered their greatness too: Galileo, Vesalius, Harvey, Morgagni. The family took Assunta from Mestre to Padua amid the Christmas rush.

The admitting physician who examined Assunta was thorough. She took an extensive family history. Assunta was obviously too sick for Meniere's disease, but it wasn't clear what she had. The doctor and her colleagues quickly came to suspect alcoholism. Assunta had all the symptoms: anxiety, sleeplessness, the shakes. Alcoholism was not publicly discussed in Italy, but that didn't mean it wasn't widespread. Shame was a huge barrier to a successful initial examination, but you couldn't let it deter you from digging out the truth. So the doctors pressed, asking Assunta over and over about her drinking habits. She said she didn't drink. The doctors pressed her again but the family insisted that Assunta was *astemia.* It was practically a fight.

The postwar boom had not made Italy a more confiding culture—many a man had left his Fascist past behind, thanks to a quiet arrangement to get hold of his party file. Deeply ingrained in the society was the assumption that any information anywhere could be used against you in ways you couldn't begin to predict. Faced with the family history portion of the admitting questionnaire, Assunta's family had put down as her father's cause of death "complications from hypertension." Pietro had had hypertension, among his other symptoms.

Assunta grew wilder at night in Padua. Sometimes the nurses tied her to the bed to keep her from rolling off. But she was not in any sort of conventional pain—no groans came from her mouth. During lucid times, she could converse normally. The doctors, stumped, performed CAT scans, PET scans, and dozens of encephalograms on her, sometimes three or four in a week, trying to peer inside her head. Her body was shaking; she was snoring loudly in her stupor. The doctors kept returning to the idea of alcoholism. Her symptoms still looked like delirium tremens to them. Only Assunta, her family said, didn't drink. But she must drink, the doctors insisted. The family didn't know how to respond. If Assunta ever drank, it was a sip of wine at dinner and the communion wine in church. "Take me away," she begged her family.

On December 30, 1973, suspecting a hidden tumor, the doctors injected dye into Assunta's arteries. While Assunta lay there, her blood pressure and her heart rate soared. The dye had caused an allergic reaction. She went into shock. The doctors performed an emergency tracheotomy and rolled her into the intensive care unit with a tube in her throat, expecting her to die, but she confounded them once more by hanging on to life.

"Tuesday he seemed better and had no fever, but then he began to worsen quickly," Assunta had written Tosca at the end of her father's life. Forty years later, Assunta had the same odd mix of symptoms. She could not walk but her comprehension was often perfect. She wasn't in pain, either. She could talk till the end, just like her father. "Whenever we asked him how he was doing, he'd say, 'Better than yesterday,' " she'd written to Tosca. "He was the one who consoled us." Assunta was the same way now. She fussed over her niece Lisi, praising her outfits or telling her not to cover her pretty face with her hair. She asked after Ignazio's medical studies. To the end, even in the midst of her immense tiredness, she was aware of where she was, who she was, what was happening to her. The day before she died, she told Lisi how pretty she looked and offered her a chocolate. The next day she died, weighing just seventy-five pounds. No longer able to swallow, she drowned in her own saliva.

Assunta had been a celebrity in the neurology ward—the tiny woman with the odd disease who wouldn't die. Her doctors wanted to do an autopsy and the family agreed. Autopsies were no longer performed in the Acquapendente, the beautiful fifteenth-century theater where the greats had studied. In the early twentieth century, the church accepted the need for postmortem examinations, which meant medical schools no longer had to hide their autopsy rooms. So officials had long since moved Padua's autopsy theater, and it was now to be found on the first floor of a modern wing of the hospital. The new facility had none of the Euclidean perfection of the old one; it was just a bright space with a long metal table and an open window to let out the smell.

Now Assunta, her body at last still, her face white in death, lay on the plain metal table. A crowd had assembled, the whole neurology department as well as curious students, Ignazio among them in the front row, in all twenty people waiting for the pathologist to prove again, as the great seventeenth-century English doctor John Sydenham had written, that it was "in the book of the dead that you discover the secrets of disease."

The pathologist first cut from the top of the sternum to the base of the belly: *il taglio cravatta,* the necktie cut. He slit open Assunta's chest and pulled out the lungs and heart, weighed them and placed them on a separate table. The lungs were heavy and when he pressed them they exuded pus, a sign of the pneumonia she had suffered from at the end. Then he sliced open Assunta's abdomen and removed her liver and her kidneys. Her liver was perfect; she had not been an alcoholic after all. But the adrenal gland on top of the kidney was atrophied. The adrenal gland is responsible for releasing adrenaline and cortisol in response to stress. The gland was burned out—it had simply given up on the demand Assunta's brain had made on it, as if, instead of lying in bed all those months or sitting at the beach or in the mountains, Assunta had been running from a pride of lions. She had been subjected to unparalleled biological stress. No one knew what to make of the finding. The professor put the organs back in the body with a good helping of sawdust and moved to the head.

The skull is amazingly strong. It is the body's citadel. The pathologist expected to find a hidden tumor somewhere in its inner workings. That had been the second theory of what made Assunta sick. So the pathologist pulled back the scalp, sawed off the skull cap, and peeled away the meninges, the fatty substances that cover the brain, lifted out the brain itself, first one hemisphere, then the other, snipping the nerves that connected it to the eyes, the carotid artery, and the spinal cord as he went. The brain was undamaged, untouched, with normal-appearing tissue. He put it on the scale. Its weight was normal, ruling out brain infection or Alzheimer's as the cause of death.

"What on earth did this woman die of?" the pathologist asked his colleagues.

"*Boh,*" one answered. "Boh" means "I don't know and I'm not likely to find out"; it is a verbal shrug. The pathologist then began to section the brain. The brain evolved from the bottom up so that when you cut down you essentially are working your way back through evolutionary time. The professor cut the brain into pieces, looking in the cerebral cortex, the midbrain, and the cerebellum for a defect he might have missed the first time. He sliced and sliced and sliced into ever finer sections, but found nothing. Proper procedure when a cause of death was not evident was to save as much of the organ as possible for later study. But the pathologist, in his frustration, kept sectioning, ruining a good portion of Assunta's brain.

On the way out, their hands still bloody, the pathologists greeted Assunta's family with another "Boh!" and then washed up. The cause of death written on Assunta's death certificate was similar to her father's: "familial encephalitis of indeterminable origin." This was another way of saying "boh."

Assunta's generation bore her death as well as they could. As they understood it, another relative had died of nervous exhaustion. They accepted that the shock of the failed relationship and menopause brought her illness on; that was still how they saw things. But Ignazio and Lisi began to ask questions. Spurred by Lisi's grandmother's comment that Assunta had the same disease as her father, she and Ignazio started piecing together the story of her family's mysterious disease. It had not paused after Pietro's death: in 1948, his sister Angela died; in 1952, his niece Luigia; in 1957, another niece, Graziella, just fourteen, supposedly of a brain tumor. In 1964 yet another young niece, Maria, who lived in Friuli, was admitted to a clinic for schizophrenia and died shortly after. Then the next year Maria's mother, Emma, died. Nineteen-sixty-five brought two more deaths among Lisi's close relatives: her cousin Rita, only twenty, and then another of Pietro's sisters, Irma, Rita's mother. Lisi, born in 1949, had known something about some of these deaths, things she began to remember. For instance, her mother had once told her about seeing Graziella asleep on top of the table in her family's house; and on the way home from Irma's funeral, Lisi, then fifteen, pretending to be asleep in the back of the car, had heard Assunta and her uncle Silvano discuss how sorrow at her daughter's death had killed Irma, and she thought to herself, even then, that no one died just of sorrow.

She also remembered that one day in 1971, when her mother went in for an operation in Venice at the same hospital at which her grandfather had died, she had snuck a peek at his chart, which the doctors had brought out. What caught her eye was similar to what had caught her mother's eye more than twenty-five years before. Then her mother had wanted to know why, if her father had encephalitis, he didn't have a headache. Now, under "spinal fluid," Lisi read the notation "clear as water in a rocky stream." (Italian medicine is full of such elegant formulations.) As a nurse, Lisi was familiar with spinal taps and thought this unlikely. The spinal fluid of encephalitis sufferers is nearly always milky colored from the immune system cells that have died fighting the infection. She told her mother and her grandmother about her find. "It's our family disease," her grandmother said matter-of-factly. "It's exhaustion." She told her not to dwell on the past. There were risks in pushing things too hard, Lisi knew. When a local doctor mentioned a "family disease," her grandmother stopped speaking to him.

Four years after Assunta's death, in the spring of 1978, Pierina, Isolina's younger sister, now in her mid-fifties, began to hold her head strangely. Her pupils shrank and she sweated. At night, she was agitated. Pierina was a typical Italian housewife, living in a nice house in Mestre. She had married after the war and, like Assunta, had never borne children, choosing to adopt one instead—perhaps she was remembering her father's death, waiting to see what would happen when she entered middle age. Pierina was an optimist, softer than Isolina and more outgoing than Assunta. Ignazio and Lisi were able to observe her more closely than they had her late sister, because they had married in 1974 and lived near Pietro's old house, where Lisi's grandmother lived. In the early stages of the disease, Pierina would come to see her aged mother, who was herself ill (though not with FFI). With the help of Lisi's mother and a cousin, Lisi and Ignazio had created a poster tracing the havoc the family disease had caused over the generations, and cut it out, appropriately, in the shape of a tree. Ignazio, now a doctor, had requested Pietro's chart from the Venice hospital and confirmed what Lisi had suspected: it was unlikely that Pietro had died of encephalitis. They felt ready, now, to confront the family mystery.

As Pierina worsened, Ignazio took control and accompanied her to see a neurologist he respected in Mestre. He told the neurologist that there was a strange inherited disease in his wife's family, that Pierina wasn't alcoholic and didn't have Alzheimer's, and that was all anyone knew. The neurologist examined Pierina and said he had no idea what was wrong with her—perhaps early Alzheimer's? So the family next took Pierina to Padua, to the same hospital that Assunta had died in almost five years before. Pierina was terrified, but the family hoped the neurologists would use the information Lisi and Ignazio had acquired since Assunta's death to help solve the family mystery. That was not to be the case. Pierina was admitted with a diagnosis of presenile dementia and went downhill quickly. Did she drink? the doctors kept asking. Did she have a tumor? They essentially gave her up for lost, weary of the puzzle the family presented. Pierina died in March 1979, weighing barely sixty-five pounds. On her death certificate the hospital put "familial encephalitis."

Again, one of Lisi's aunts was the center of attention in the autopsy theater. Again the pathologist threw up his hands. This time, the brain was sealed in paraffin for later study. Soon after, Ignazio took it on a train to see a famous neurologist in Geneva, Dr. Johannes Wildi, who held the post of neurological consultant for the hospitals of Europe. Wildi greeted Ignazio with slides at the ready and together they mounted some tissue and looked at Pierina's brain under a micro-scope. Nothing looked out of order. Ignazio left the brain and went home. Wildi promised to send him a more detailed analysis of the tis-sue and Ignazio got back a five-page letter two weeks later in which Wildi noted that the main damage in Pierina's head was to the thala-mus—part of it had nearly been destroyed—but, he added, he could not figure out what the connection was between that fact and the symp-toms Ignazio had described. The only disease he could think of as a candidate was Alzheimer's. Ignazio wrote back that he did not think Pierina could have had Alzheimer's but, having observed her loss of coordination and dementia, he thought perhaps the family disease might have something in common with Creutzfeldt-Jakob disease. Ig-nazio was already becoming a gifted clinician—if the answer wasn't the obvious he went back and thought again. Wildi responded that the tiny holes in the brain he saw did resemble the holes seen in Creutzfeldt-Jakob disease, but that, since CJD did not attack the thala-mus, it could not be the correct diagnosis.

Wildi asked whether there were any more brains from the family he could examine, so Ignazio wrote to the hospital in Padua to get the cat-alog number for the pieces of Assunta's brain that had been preserved. He sent the number to Wildi, who consulted his own catalogue of Ital-ian pathological tissue (Wildi's file cabinets held some of the most baf-fling tissue in Italy). Wildi said Assunta was not among his holdings. He mentioned to Ignazio that one of the doctors who'd been at the au-topsy used to work for him and had a reputation for walking off with in-teresting body parts. Did he have the sections of Assunta's brain? That man was now a neurologist in another country, and when Ignazio ap-proached him, he wrote back that he had no idea what Ignazio was talk-ing about.

Neither Wildi nor Ignazio was shocked. Interesting cases were valuable. Brain tissue was constantly "going missing" in this era. Per-haps the man had seen something interesting and decided not to let the opportunity to get a better look slip away. He had done this quietly, informally, risking jail, to avoid the red tape that might have made the thing legal but probably would have made it impossible. The pieces of Assunta's brain had simply gone into his pocket.

One can imagine him, this young man, worried about the unreliable electricity in a time of shortages, pulling pieces of Assunta's brain out from time to time with increasing frustration, slicing them thin, fixing them to slides, and putting them under his microscope, trying to connect the tiny pinpricks in the thalamus to the panoply of known human neurological diseases, hopeful of making a find that would enshrine his name in medical history for all time.

CHAPTER 8

A WONDERFUL PROBLEM FOR A CHEMIST

SAN FRANCISCO, *late 1970s to early 1980s*

The problem, when Stanley Prusiner entered what Carleton Gajdusek named the "slow virus" field in 1974, was the one Gajdusek left it with: no one had proven what the infectious agent behind scrapie, kuru, and Creutzfeldt-Jakob disease was. It could be a virus, it could be a protein, it could be a combination of the two, or it could be something else entirely. Before it could be properly identified, someone was going to have to separate it from the material that surrounded it in tissue and look at it under an electron microscope or by means of X-ray crystallography. Infectious disease specialists, though, thought the level of purification necessary to retrieve something so small would be too hard and too expensive to achieve. Prusiner disagreed.

A deliberate man with extraordinary drive, Prusiner first realized slow viruses were a problem he wanted to explore when he saw a CJD patient in a hospital in 1972, soon after he graduated from medical school. He read the history of the attempts to identify the cause of scrapie and Tikvah Alper's remarkable experiments that showed the agent could not be destroyed by radiation and became convinced that a protein without DNA was behind the disease. His comments were met with skepticism by mainstream scientists; the rejection made him mad, and the anger made him focus even more.

Prusiner was in many ways the opposite of Gajdusek. In high school, he was turned down for the advanced chemistry class. "He basically goofed off," remembered a high school friend. Whereas Gajdusek went to Rochester, Caltech, and Harvard Medical School, three renowned institutions, Prusiner attended the University of Pennsylvania and the U. Penn. medical school, a notch below. No quartet of Nobel Prize winners ushered him through his early training, as they had Gajdusek, nor did he have Gajdusek's gift for seeking them out.

Prusiner first set to work on slow viruses in the mid-1970s in collaboration with William Hadlow, the veterinary pathologist who had pointed out to Gajdusek the parallels between kuru and scrapie. Hadlow's operation was a massive one. His fifteen-person group injected, by his estimate, ten thousand mice, a thousand mink, and a hundred to a hundred and fifty sheep and goats in a crawl to understand more about the agent. Prusiner watched impatiently from his University of California–San Francisco office, from which he supplied some of the innoculant Hadlow used. In the late 1970s, the NIH grew frustrated and cut off its funding for the project. All the animals were euthanized. Prusiner too looked like a casualty of the scrapie mystery.

Gajdusek was on the fence about the nature of the slow virus particle. He was not really a lab scientist; he was more of a clinician—and the molecular world did not excite him. But Prusiner was comfortable in the world of reagents and centrifuges. He brought a number of skills to the investigation that Gajdusek lacked, skills that hinted he might get further than his predecessor. As he pointed out in a 1986 article, the slow virus agent "had been attacked by pathologists, physicians, veterinarians, [but] it became clear that this was a wonderful problem for a chemist," which Prusiner was. Chemists specialized in separating tiny quantities of matter from other tiny quantities; they were meticulous. Prusiner was also technically inventive, finding clever shortcuts for the field. For instance, he substituted hamsters for mice in his lab experiments: hamsters got sick a lot faster. In 1984, he bragged that he had sped up the work of purifying the scrapie protein a hundredfold. Such efficiency was not the sort of thing anyone could imagine Gajdusek caring about.

Prusiner knew that the way to figure out the nature of the scrapie particle was to get rid of everything else in the gunk around it. You had to keep stripping away molecules until you were left with the ones that were actually responsible for the infection. The process consists of taking syringes full of infection tissue and shooting them into animals, then killing the animals once they get sick and putting their brain tissue into a centrifuge and spinning it fast enough for the molecules to separate. Then you take the separated-out molecules and inject them into mice or hamsters. If some get sick quicker than others, you know that they received a more concentrated agent: you keep repeating the process until you've come as close to purity as possible. Then you try to define the agent by its properties. Does it dissolve in water? What dye does it react with? And so on.

Paradoxically, the purification of something as small as a protein is a commitment to scale. From 1975 to 1997, the NIH gave Prusiner $56 million in grants and he used some of it to fill his lab with scores of post-docs and researchers to work on slow viruses. It was a project that devoured time, money, and mice. But Prusiner began to make progress. By the mid-1980s, Prusiner wrote that he had separated out an agent five thousand times more concentrated than that which occurred naturally. The agent was now pure enough to measure, and

Prusiner and his colleagues found it was small even for a protein and much smaller than the smallest known viruses. They then began to tease out its biochemical qualities. They tried mixing the agent with enzymes that dissolve proteins and with enzymes that dissolve nucleic acid. They found that chemicals that destroyed proteins destroyed the particle's infectivity, whereas chemicals that destroyed nucleic acids actually increased the infectivity; this information gave a strong hint that the infection resided in a protein and not in a virus. With a highly purified agent now in its possession, Prusiner's lab was also able to design an antibody to react to it. This advance made it possible to test for the presence of the infectious agent simply by taking some of a victim's tissue and exposing it to the antibody. If the antibody reacted, you knew the animal had a scrapie infection. The era of endless inoculations and years of waiting was over: there was now a cheaper, faster way to see whether a person had CJD or a sheep scrapie than taking his brain tissue and injecting it into animals.

Prusiner chronicled his progress in a succession of papers in science journals. Those papers don't make exciting reading; they are like postcards from a traveler who writes to you from every local train stop, extending little by little what he can say with confidence about the view out the window.

But if Prusiner was cautious in his science, he was often reckless in his relationships with other scientists. The anger that had propelled him into prion research did not make him easy to work with or supportive of his staff. His haughtiness offended other scrapie researchers, who had come to think of their specialty as a club of the long-suffering. And, like many who belong to clubs, scrapie researchers were more aware of their own efforts than of larger movements outside them. Prusiner broke the club's rules in a lot of ways. He was stingy in acknowledging the sources of his ideas: he wanted the field to begin and end with him. He seemed convinced that he had originated the idea that there might be an infectious agent that did not contain any

DNA. He forgot that the theory began with the English mathematician J. S. Griffith; that British researchers had brought the theory a certain distance forward, and Gajdusek had carried it further still. "Repeat and expand and the original will never be cited again. That's Stan's trick," says Gajdusek's former colleague Paul Brown of the NIH.

Protein and virology labs are full of Prusiner's former graduate students who, mysteriously, left the prion field once they left Prusiner's lab. "I've had people tell me that he told them that they'd better not go into competition with him or he'd ruin them," says Richard Johnson, a longtime friend of Prusiner's who is a microbiologist at Johns Hopkins University.

Prusiner has also thrown his weight around in the peer review process. When a researcher submits a paper for publication in a scientific journal, the journal's editors give it to other scientists in the same field to judge its accuracy and significance. In effect, one's competitors are also one's judges. This system works only if scientists put their interest in truth ahead of their ambition, and most scientists do, but Prusiner, in the mid-1980s, was asked by *The New England Journal of Medicine* to judge a paper submitted by Paul Brown. Prusiner recommended that the *NEJM* reject it and then submitted a similar one based on his lab's work (the *NEJM* ultimately published Brown's and turned down Prusiner's). Years of crossed swords have left their mark on the field. At prion conferences, all eyes are on Prusiner with his styled tuft of white hair: half the room hopes to gain his notice and the other half quietly curses him.

Prusiner is in many ways more a manager than an investigator: he assembles talented staffs and runs them hard. A former researcher of his—like most, unwilling to let his name be used—dismisses his old boss as "the general contractor of prion research." But is that such a bad thing? One way Prusiner keeps prion science advancing is through his gift for getting grants; research money is the life's blood of science today, and in 2001, Prusiner's lab was the top recipient of NIH funds in the country. He has more drive than anyone else in the field and more perspective, and he understands where prion research must go in ways that others do not. He is a scientist beautifully adapted to the present day, when the academic scientist who lives on collegial accolades and university largesse has given way to the entrepreneurial researcher who forms alliances in politics and business to keep his work, and, sometimes, his business ventures, going.

At times Prusiner seems to confuse the two. In 2000, he founded a company called InPro Biotechnology that markets a test for prion disease. Soon he was pressing Congress to require testing of every slaughtered American cow. His implication that beef might be unsafe in America was particularly glaring because in 1997, before he had a test to sell, he told the press after he won the Nobel Prize that he was going to celebrate by eating a T-bone steak, the riskiest kind of beef because it contains a piece of the spine, where prions accumulate.

Prusiner likes to make money and spend it, living well on a half-million-dollar salary from the medical school of the University of California at San Francisco. He wants the best bottle of wine and the biggest house with the biggest pool when he travels. The divorce papers filed by his wife in 2000 mention their patronizing "the best restaurants" and buying "expensive art" and "fashionable clothes." (Prusiner responded that he had only lived lavishly during the Nobel Prize ceremony, and at others' expense.) Prusiner is at home in the world of conferences, luxury hotels, and business-class air travel, not in the field Gajdusek loved. When he visited New Guinea to examine kuru firsthand in the late 1970s, Prusiner quickly wore himself out in the bush. "He was so exhausted it was hard to tell if he had sprained something or was just too tired to walk," remembered Michael Alpers, who runs the kuru research program in Okapa.

Gajdusek was appalled, at a party at Prusiner's house, to find all anyone talked about was schools and country clubs, the very stuff Gajdusek had fled to New Guinea to avoid. To add insult to injury,

Prusiner had furnished his home with statues he had bought in New Guinea, their genitals removed for decency—or so Gajdusek remembers. The two men do not criticize each other in public, but Gajdusek thinks Prusiner is a derivative thinker, and Prusiner thinks Gajdusek is undisciplined. "I think Stan's feeling is that when you look at what Gajdusek actually did scientifically, his contribution was minimal at best," says a scientist who knows them both well. According to this man, Prusiner believes that Gajdusek took the idea for his key experiment from William Hadlow, the scrapie researcher; that Michael Alpers in Papua New Guinea did the fieldwork; and that C. J. Gibbs, Gajdusek's lab director, did the transmission work, with Gajdusek mostly showing up to claim the credit. Meanwhile, Gajdusek claims—inaccurately—that Prusiner trained with him. Both are ambitious, but their ambition is expressed through different temperaments. "Carleton's an egoist, Stan's an egotist," says Paul Brown of the NIH.

In the early 1980s, Prusiner realized that Gajdusek's "slow virus" terminology was holding the field back in the crucial realm of public awareness. Before the early twentieth century, "virus" was a generic term for an infectious agent, but modern scientists understood it to mean, specifically, a core of DNA or RNA coated by protein. And the label "transmissible viral spongiform encephalopathy"—used by Gajdusek and others to describe the diseases scrapie, kuru, and CJD—also fell short in Prusiner's eyes. For one thing, not all the infections were transmissible; possibly, none were viral; and you didn't always find sponginess in the victim's brain (sometimes you found plaques). But the biggest problem with the term was that no one could remember it.

Prusiner knew he had to give a new name to whatever it was he was closing in on. In a story he likes to tell, an astrophysicist friend advised him to choose a term that was as memorable as "quark," something simple and striking. Prusiner mulled it over, passing the time at boring meetings making acrostics of contenders. Eventually, he came up with "prion." *Nature* called it "a rather tortured acronym of 'small proteinaceous infectious particle.' " Tortured, perhaps, but memorable. "Prion" made biochemistry sexy, because it sounded cutting edge, as if a physicist had discovered it: electron, neutron, photon . . . prion. Prusiner's friends thought part of the appeal to him of the word "prion" was that the sound was reminiscent of his own name.

Prusiner told his colleagues how happy he was with his coinage. The word did have a preexisting meaning: a prion was a flightless bird found in the South Seas, "a fluttering thing of pale grey-blue and white . . . a ghost," as one magazine described it. Elio Lugaresi, an Italian sleep researcher who co-discovered fatal familial insomnia, re- counts Prusiner's telling the story of looking in a new dictionary a few years after he'd debuted prion, the infectious agent, to see whether "his" prion was now listed ahead of prion, the bird. He noticed that the avian prion had dropped out altogether. " 'I think it's extinct,' " Prusiner exclaimed with delight.

To Prusiner's opponents, the real offense of his actions was that "proteinaceous infectious particle," out of which "prion" somewhat illogically derives, avoided the key question in the field: was the infec- tious agent a protein or a virus? Not even Prusiner knew the answer. He seemed to be trying to solve a scientific dispute with a verbal trick. They felt he'd put the cart before the horse. Many researchers refused to go along for the ride. Some took to using the redundant phrase "prion protein," demoting Prusiner's noun to an adjective to remove the implication that he had discovered a new disease principle. They preferred a vocabulary that left open the possibility that the disease lay in an associated infectious nucleic acid, something more like a virus. In Britain, researchers pronounce what Prusiner calls a *"pree-*on" a *"pry-*on," an assertion of independence in the face of another Ameri- can invasion.

Prusiner's audacity has been the object of many jokes in the lab. One, a limerick by an anonymous researcher, goes:

There was a young turk named Stan
Who embarked on a devious plan.
"If I simply rename it, I'm sure I can claim it,"
Said Stan as he pondered his scam.

"Eureka!" cried Stan, "I have found it.
Well . . . maybe not actually found it.
But I talked to the press
Of the slow virus mess
And invented a name to confound it!"

Yet the word "prion" enthralled the press, just as Prusiner had hoped. His hometown paper, the *San Francisco Chronicle,* broke the news of the "discovery" of the prion on its front page. The headline was "Tiny Life Form Found." Newspapers emphasized the toughness of the prion, how heat and radiation could do nothing to destroy it, and the way once land was infected with prions it was always infected. The *Chronicle* mentioned that not even rattlesnake or cobra venom could kill a prion. The press had always loved kuru. Now they had an infectious agent as intriguing as the disease it caused.

Prusiner knew what he had to do to silence skeptics: synthesize a prion in a test tube and make it cause a prion disease. Then no one could say there was a virus hiding behind the protein, doing the dirty work of infection. But prions had a surprise in store for Prusiner. Once he and his lab purified the prion enough to determine part of its amino acid sequence, they were shocked to find that prions were ordinary proteins manufactured by a healthy gene in the host's own body. In other words, prions were not something that infected the victim from outside; they were something the victim himself produced.

This revelation could not be squared with what prion researchers thought they knew: that prions caused infection. How could a gene cause an infection in its own host? It cast in doubt all the time, money, and intellectual energy Prusiner and everyone else had invested in prions.

Shortly after, in an alliance with two other research labs, Prusiner announced that he had found the gene that made the prion. It was on Chromosome 20, among what would turn out to be seven hundred or so other genes, including genes that control insulin production, weight gain, and childhood eczema. The prion gene makes the prion through the same process by which the body manufactures all proteins: by creating a blueprint of amino acids that another part of the cell, called the ribosome, then puts into manufacture. How could the ordinary protein-manufacturing process hold if prions were infectious? Researchers hoped to find an answer by figuring out the role normal prions played in the body, but what they would learn was not illuminating. If they eliminated the prion gene in mice, the mice did fine. Yet the gene had to do something, because all mammals turned out to have it. Genes persist only when they have a function. Here was a gene that appeared to create a protein that had no function except to make its possessor sick. There had to be something wrong with the idea: it flew in the face of all the laws of adaptation and evolution.

A new theory, one that allowed for a deadly protein produced by the victim's own body, had to enter the picture. Prusiner had once suggested that prions, when they entered the body, were able to deconstruct themselves, converting their amino acids back into the DNA that had originally specified their manufacture. Then, in theory, the DNA would reverse gears to produce multiple copies of the infectious agent. It was a beautiful scenario; the only problem was that there was no example of it in nature. In any event, the discovery of the prion gene made this proposal obsolete, though without leaving anything to replace it. No one knew how a normal protein could produce diseased copies of itself. Finally, Prusiner suggested a possibility straight out of chemistry, rather than biology: infection by means of a protein template. He posited that prions had two forms, one infectious, one not. If an infectious protein came into contact with a normal one, it bound to it, causing it to change shape into a copy of the infectious one. The idea was originally that of the English mathematician J. S. Griffith, and fifteen years after he first proposed it, it still invited the same objection, as Prusiner well knew it would: no one had ever seen a protein behave in this way. It was simply not what proteins did.

Yet it seemed they must, if Prusiner's data—and those coming from a lot of other researchers—were correct. In the mid-1980s, Prusiner tried to clinch the protein-only hypothesis by creating prions in a test tube using the newly found prion gene and injecting them into mice. Had the experiment worked, it would have proven that prions and prions alone caused disease, but the obstacle that Prusiner ran into was that the normal prion gene did not make much prion and that which it made was the healthy, nondeformed kind. The mice did not get sick. It looked as if those researchers who insisted prions without nucleic acids were harmless might be right. But then Prusiner and his staff realized that they didn't have to design an experiment to show that prions cause illness, because nature had already done so.

There was by now a lot of evidence that prion diseases were inherited. CJD was no longer the "dumping ground" diagnosis it had been. After Prusiner and other researchers developed an antibody to the prion in the early 1980s, neurologists had a fast, reliable way to distinguish prion diseases from brain diseases with similar symptoms, such as Pick's disease and Alzheimer's. And once the prion gene was found, researchers had little trouble finding mutations on it that caused the various inherited prion diseases. Both inherited CJD and inherited Gerstmann-Sträussler-Scheinker disease (GSS) were now established diagnoses. In the late 1980s, Prusiner realized that these genetic prion diseases might supply a backdoor proof that prions caused infection. He put genes with prion disease–causing mutations in them into mice and then when the mice got sick, he killed them, took the infectious prions from them and injected them into new mice without the mutation. Some of these mice, too, got sick. Prusiner called this the "persuasive experiment."

It was close to proof that prions cause prion disease, because the mice had not been exposed to an infection, only to the deformed proteins of a defective gene. But the experiment left open the possibility that prions didn't cause the disease but simply altered the body in a way that allowed viruses already in the body to become lethal. Gajdusek particularly had been interested in viruses that stayed inert for decades until activated by alterations in the body's own chemistry, like the viruses that cause warts. A similar virus could be causing GSS or CJD, with prions just preparing the way.

Opponents of the protein-only theory hammered on this possibility. Where, Prusiner responded, was this ubiquitous virus, then? It hadn't shown up in any purification, and the purified prion was now so small that, if there was a nucleic acid hiding in it, it wouldn't be enough to code a virus. The protein-virus debate had become a standoff between a proven mechanism—viral infection—and lab evidence that there was only a protein.

Actually, neither the protein-only theory nor the viral theory quite explained the many ways prions could cause disease. It was clear that prion disease could be genetic. That idea did not present any intellectual challenge. There were many genetic protein diseases. Gajdusek had also already shown that prion disease could be infectious, at least when prions were injected into animals. But there was a third prion disease scenario, and that one was odder. In some cases, a single individual came down with Creutzfeldt-Jakob disease. Yet no one else in his or her family had symptoms, and neither did any descendants. On examination, their prion genes turned out to be normal, but one could inject tissue from the victim into mice and the mice would get sick. These victims tended to be old; beyond that the disease just seemed to strike at random. The medical term for this sort of disease pattern is "sporadic." In all of medicine, there was no example of a single disease that could be sporadic, infectious, and genetic the way Creutzfeldt-Jakob disease appeared to.

The solution to this puzzle, according to Prusiner, could be found in the nature of proteins. The body manufactures proteins in the form of long strings, but they almost immediately begin to bend and pleat and tuck themselves elaborately in preparation for their functions in the cell. Although a given protein may well have many possible forms, usually only one form is stable. If you force a different shape on a protein, it will bounce back to whatever state its molecular bonds allow it to be most stable in.

The prion is unusual in that it seems to have two naturally occurring normal forms: two ways of staying folded. Sometimes the prion can be found in one state, sometimes in the other. In the first state, the prion fulfills its normal (unknown) function in the cell. In the second state, the prion causes prion disease. When a disease-causing prion is placed with a normal prion in a test tube, the diseased one can sometimes convert the normal one to the former's shape.

Here, then, was a theory broad enough to explain all prion infections. Disease-causing prions spread by getting other prion proteins with which they come into contact to shift shapes and become like them, in a process called conformational influence. Conformational influence can explain the various forms of prion diseases. In inherited cases, a genetic mutation causes a defect in the makeup of the protein, which causes the protein to fold badly, in turn deforming adjacent proteins. In sporadic cases, a first protein misfolds by chance, and then sets off a chain reaction. In infectious cases, such as kuru, a misfolded protein from an outside source comes into contact with the host's normal proteins and causes them to misfold. The explanation is powerful enough to make even scrapie explicable. The reason the epidemiological patterns of scrapie baffled shepherds and veterinarians over two centuries was that there were really three ways sheep might get scrapie: they inherited it (or at least inherited a very strong susceptibility to it), they contracted it from other sheep or from contaminated land, or they got it by chance.

Conformational influence as a way to pass on information usually conveyed with DNA seemed a revolutionary idea, but in fact it was a throwback. The idea of a molecule that other molecules use as a template had been the orthodoxy when the belief that proteins controlled reproduction was in its heyday, before James Watson and Francis Crick's revelations about the structure of DNA established how DNA conveyed genetic information. Among those who'd believed in molecular templates passionately were Carleton Gajdusek's own teachers, the Nobel laureates Max Delbrück and Linus Pauling. As the evidence had increased that DNA was the key to replication, authorities like Delbrück and Pauling had objected. The idea that genetic information might be conveyed through a set of chemical compounds—nucleic acids—that existed only for that purpose seemed, to use Robert Bakewell's term of opprobrium, "unthrifty." They blamed the DNA hypothesis on faulty lab techniques. Similarly, researchers who now still think a virus is hiding alongside the prion protein insist that lab purification techniques simply haven't reached the level of sensitivity necessary to find the culprit. They dub prion science the "cold fusion" of biology and say time is on their side. They point out that purification is not a cheap process; and with Prusiner controlling so much of the money in the field, they do not have the resources to test out their theories. Prion advocates respond that for a bit of infectious nucleic acid to be so tiny they still haven't found it, you'd have to invent a doctrine even more radical than theirs. (James Watson does not agree. Now almost eighty and the head of the Cold Spring Harbor Laboratory, he says that the molecular mechanism by which prions supposedly replicate have yet to be worked out to his satisfaction. Prions, in his view, remain "a mystery.")

Many researchers in the prion field are, as Paul Brown of the NIH puts it, "agnostic" on the prion theory. Their experiments don't depend on the nature of the infectious molecule; it is enough for them to know that a protein plays an important part in the prion disease process. Stop the protein from converting other proteins and you have a good chance to stop the disease. Prusiner himself has developed a more complex theory of prions over the years. He now believes there is another protein of unknown shape and size—with characteristic showmanship, he calls it protein X—that helps the normal prion shift shape to the defective one. There are tens of thousands of proteins in a human cell, many of which help other proteins to maintain or change their forms; one may well perform this function.

The gold standard to prove that prions cause infection is still to make a prion in a test tube and then inject it into a lab animal that then gets a prion disease. For twenty years, Prusiner's lab and others tried this experiment. Then in July 2004, Prusiner's lab announced success. Briefly, the Holy Grail seemed in his hands. "We have compelling evidence," he told *The New York Times*. "We've done it all." Not so fast, prion skeptics and Prusiner's detractors (by now practically one and the same) said. It turned out Prusiner had bred the mice with souped-up prion genes, which allowed the mice to get sick from far less prion protein than would be necessary under natural conditions. The mice were in fact so primed to get prion disease that some developed it *without* an injection. Prusiner's lab responded that they were working on a proof using ordinary mice. Alan Dickinson, the scrapie researcher at Scotland's Moredun Institute and a prion skeptic, claims a friend has a manuscript debunking the whole prion hypothesis just waiting for the day researchers find the nucleic acid behind prion diseases. Meanwhile, the dust thickens on the title page.

CHAPTER 9

CONVERGENCE THE VENETO, *1983*

If I can make it past 55, I've got it made.

— S I L V A N O , aged fifty-three

The Italian family didn't know about the controversy over the nature of the prion agent. They didn't know about the discoveries in the
prion field going on at the NIH, in Britain, and in San Francisco from
the 1960s through the early 1980s, and Carleton Gajdusek, Stanley
Prusiner, and their colleagues had never heard of the Italian family.
The suggestion made by Ignazio, and seconded by Johannes Wildi, the
great Swiss neurologist, after Pierina's death in 1979 that the family
disease looked like CJD lay fallow. There was no one with the background, skills, or knowledge to pursue it.

Pierina's death was followed by a period of calm. Lisi and Ignazio
did not hear of any relatives who had suddenly lost the ability to sleep.
But obviously, Pietro's three remaining children—Isolina and Tosca,
both in their late fifties, and Silvano, in his late forties—remained at

risk. Lisi, now in her late twenties, became obsessive about whether she would get the disease too. She knew that her fate would be made clearer by what happened to her mother, so she followed Isolina around the house day and night, and any time her mother had insomnia, Lisi panicked. "I was a spy in my own house," she recalled. "I'd sneak up to her room and make sure she was really asleep." During these "years lived in hell," Lisi herself began to suffer insomnia and grew afraid she was falling victim to FFI. She and Ignazio held off having children, because, until her mother was out of danger, they were not going to take the risk that they would be adding yet another chapter to the family's miserable story.

In the summer of 1983, Silvano, Lisi's uncle, was living with Isolina in the house they grew up in. Silvano had recently been held at gunpoint during a bank robbery in Venice. Shortly after, he had gone on a cruise with his mother, when for the first time he'd been ashamed to dance, his shirt was so sweaty. Now he looked in the mirror and saw his pupils were small as pinpricks and he was holding his head stiffly. The proteins that would bring about his end were beginning the deadly process of malforming. He did not know this, of course—no one did yet. All he knew was that soon he would stop sleeping and what would come next. "If I can make it past fifty-five, I've got it made," he'd told a childhood friend for years. He was fifty-three.

Silvano was a handsome man with the red hair of his great-grandmother Marianna, a strong brow, and a trim frame. With his graceful movements and elegant appearance, a pocket square always folded in his jacket, he could easily have been mistaken for a movie star. He loved movies, too, especially the poise its stars showed. Attractive to women, he never told his girlfriends about his fears that he would die young. For Silvano, intimacy was what you reserved for your family. He was very devoted to them; to Lisi, whose own father was disabled, he fulfilled much of the parental role. He also served as a bridge to the richer parts of the family, the branches not afflicted by the disease. He had learned the social formulas that would allow him access to a grander world than his father had lived in. He made money and spent it, as if he believed in his heart there was no reason to save for old age.

Silvano was not going to go the way his sisters had gone. He was not going to allow curious doctors to torment him. For as long as he could, he would stay out of their hands. As his afternoon nap disappeared and his night sleep dwindled, he tried to use his insomnia to his advantage, working harder and staying out later. Finally, in February 1984, Lisi's husband, Ignazio, persuaded him to come with him to see a neurologist in Castelfranco, a small city in the northwestern Veneto. The neurologist diagnosed anxiety and depression and gave Silvano some Halcion, a sedative. The next night Isolina called Ignazio to come see what had happened. Silvano was at the bottom of the stairs, packing an imaginary suitcase. He tried to sleepwalk out the door but couldn't get it unlocked. Ignazio discontinued the drug.

Remarkably, nine months after his first symptoms, Silvano was still working. He cut back his social life; otherwise he continued living as before. It helped that he had to spend a lot of time traveling—he worked for a company that ran public sector construction projects—so his colleagues couldn't observe him too closely. Only his sleep would not cooperate. It was growing lighter and lighter, and he was sweating relentlessly. Still, under no circumstances was he going to go to Padua, where his two sisters had died.

In March, Ignazio convinced Silvano to come to the hospital in Treviso where Ignazio was now an internist. Ignazio told his superior he had an interesting case of familial encephalitis; could he please have a bed? The neurologist from Castelfranco came for a consultation with the head of neurology at Treviso and could not believe Silvano was the same man he had seen a month before, he seemed so much weaker. "What's he got?" the neurologist asked Ignazio. "He's got a total insomnia," Ignazio said. The two neurologists had a good laugh: total insomnia was impossible. Sleep was a homeostatic function; eventually the body corrected the deficit. It had to, or else the patient would die, and as everyone knew, no one ever died from lack of sleep. From then on, Ignazio told people that his mysterious patient was demented, and the staff left him and Silvano alone.

Because Ignazio was not a neurologist, he had no preconceptions about what might be causing his wife's family disease. He ran every test he could think of on his wife's uncle, but except for the extraordinarily high level of a few hormones, none of the results seemed out of the ordinary. One Sunday, when there was no one around, he asked a friendly technician to run a long electroencephalograph on Silvano. Normally EEGs are snapshots; they last a minute. Ignazio wanted a half hour's worth, a filmstrip of Silvano's brain activity. "Do me a favor," he said, "use up thirty feet of paper on this one."

What he saw was unprecedented: Silvano's brain waves went up and down in a fast, jagged pattern that did not correspond to either sleep or wakefulness and that did not exist in the medical literature. He was living in some sort of in-between world. Ignazio thought if he could only break this pattern for an hour, Silvano's systems might come back into balance. He toyed with the idea of giving him general anesthesia, but remembered the side effects of the Halcion. He was stumped. One day he mentioned the strange case of his wife's uncle to an eye doctor friend, who said that the man who knew most about sleep was Elio Lugaresi, the director of the sleep clinic at the University of Bologna. Since Silvano's problem seemed to involve a disturbance of sleep, Ignazio should get in contact with him.

Elio Lugaresi had entered the field of sleep study in the early 1960s, when it was almost new. It had been an adventurous decision, because until the middle of the twentieth century, sleep had barely been studied. Doctors assumed that nothing happened during sleep, much as nothing happened during a coma: the brain shut down and rested. Anyone watching a sleeping person closely—the irregular breathing, the nictitating eyelids, the periodic body movements—could have disputed this portrait, but sitting up all night watching a person asleep required more commitment than most doctors had. Besides, sleep had its seat in the brain and the brain was a black box.

In the 1930s a small bit of progress was made. Researchers began to use EEG machines to record brain waves. In 1953, a Chicago researcher named Nathaniel Kleitman, using an EEG, discovered rapid eye movement (REM) sleep. What was interesting about REM sleep was that EEGs showed the brain was as active during this period as when awake. Suddenly, the idea of sleep as a kind of mini-death was out, and the nocturnal eight hours became a new and varied landscape.

There things more or less stopped. Even in the 1980s researchers were still scratching at the surface of sleep: they now knew that sleep began with rough alpha waves, then deepened into longer theta waves, which were followed by sleep spindles, which took the sleeper into the profound sleep of the rolling delta wave, which itself was broken periodically by the hectic interruption of REM sleep. But sleep researchers remained more tourists than authorities on the body's nighttime voyage, longer on descriptions than on explanations. All the same, Lugaresi liked his work and was good at it, becoming known internationally for his subtle reading of the EEG printouts his sleep lab produced and, within Italy, for his ability to shake loose funding from the bureaucracy.

This latter skill was particularly impressive, because whereas in northern European nations sleep studies were a part of the national fabric, sleeplessness was not a very Italian problem—in fact the language has no easy word for it. People who can't sleep speak of *"una notte in bianco,"* a night in white, a term that only dates from the 1900s. In recent years, however, Italy, having joined the modern, industrialized world, had begun to experience the modern world's psychological problems in earnest. By the 1970s, millions of Italians had sleep problems. Lugaresi, charming and persuasive and a committed leftist in the city known as "Red Bologna," capitalized on the boom in "*lo stress*": his university bought him state-of-the-art EEG machines that even the Americans admired. And when Ignazio called him and asked if the professor had time to see his wife's uncle, Lugaresi told the family to come the next day.

Lugaresi met Silvano, Ignazio, and Lisi in his office in the Neurological Institute at the northern end of the arcaded city. The Institute is in a gray late-nineteenth-century building, Venetian in style on top and Florentine below. In the 1920s it had been a clinic for victims of Von Economo's disease. Lugaresi was struck by this handsome, broad-shouldered man in front of him. He responded to his cultivation and knew they both understood and cared about the art of living. (The only time I saw Lugaresi truly upset was when, after taking me to a restaurant that specialized in wine, he found out I didn't drink it; and the happiest I saw him was on a winter's day a year later when we were at a restaurant and the proprietor honored him with a perfect truffle to take home.)

A young neurologist named Pietro Cortelli took Silvano's admission information. He asked Silvano what was wrong with him, and Silvano answered him simply, "I am going to die. I've watched my father die and my two sisters die from the same disease that's been in our family for generations. I can tell you exactly how I will go."

He asked for a day to tell his story. He told Cortelli about the family, how for the past century and a half they'd left an eerie record of premature demise, of the parish books full of the family's odd deaths. The latest to die was his sister Pierina. He was next. Cortelli tried to comfort Silvano. The young physician was by nature optimistic, and anyone who entered the bleak field of neurology quickly learned the art of euphemism. "There are cures and therapies we can give you," he said.

"Let's not waste time in such nonsense," Silvano answered. "I assume you'll want the brain when it's time?"

Silvano was given a room with a comfortable bed. He was calm and resigned. When a friend from childhood came to see him, he told him: "Well, finally we're here." A videotape machine was set up to record his behavior, and his head was covered with sensors connected to an EEG machine. Lugaresi, Cortelli, and their staff observed from another room.

The perverse pathology of fatal familial insomnia, as his family's disease would come to be called, moves the imagination, even of scientists. Pierluigi Gambetti, the co-discoverer of FFI, says that the Italian family reminds him of the sleepless townspeople of Macondo, frozen in their "state of hallucinated lucidity," in Gabriel García Márquez's *One Hundred Years of Solitude.* But watching the tapes in Lugaresi's lab, more than fifteen years after Silvano died, I kept thinking of the stories of Edgar Allan Poe, in which the boundary between consciousness, sleep, and death is menacingly blurred. In particular, there is Poe's "Facts in the Case of M. Valdemar," in which a doctor tells the story of a patient who, though without vital signs, can still respond through hypnosis to questions.

As Silvano knew it would be, his course was relentlessly downward. On a tape made in March 1984, his eyelids flutter over the dots of his eyes. Already, as in "M. Valdemar," the "glassy roll of the eye was changed for that expression of uneasy inward examination which is never seen except in cases of sleep-walking." During good moments, Silvano could still read. He wore his glasses on the end of his nose. He ticked off the days on a pad so he wouldn't get disoriented. He dressed in black silk pajamas with a pocket square and continued to receive visitors.

The nights were not so smooth. At night, Silvano dreamed, reenacting memories of his old life, just as his sisters had. FFI strips its sufferers not just physically but psychologically. Silvano had always loved social life. He had even found the old crest of the Venetian doctor—black and red with a gold star—and hung it outside his bedroom. Now, in his dreams, Silvano carefully combed his hair, as if for a party. Once he saluted as if he were part of the changing guard at Buckingham Palace. He picked an orchid and offered it to the Queen of England.

During lucid moments, Silvano could laugh with Ignazio and Lisi over what was happening—he joked that the brain-sensor cap on his head made him look like Celestine V, and that, like the thirteenth-century pope, he wanted to renounce his crown—but such joking did not disguise his terror. Two months into his stay at Bologna, he was howling in the night, his arms and legs wrapped around themselves, the tiny pocket square still in place. In the last days of his life he lay in a twitchy, exhausted nothingness. "Are you dead?" the doctor asks Valdemar at the end of Poe's story. Valdemar's response is chilling: "For God's sake quick!—quick!—put me to sleep—or, quick!—waken me!—quick!—I say to you that I am dead!" That was Silvano.

After three months at the clinic, there was one more torment in store for him: clinic rules prohibited patients from remaining indefi-nitely unless they were in the final stages of life. Ignazio assured the clinic that his wife's uncle would be dead soon, but he had no real evi-dence for his prognosis. So Silvano had to go back to Treviso, where Ig-nazio was a doctor, by ambulance, until Cortelli, the young neurologist who had interviewed him, intervened and brought him back. Two weeks later, just as Ignazio had predicted, Silvano was dead.

As Silvano had weakened, Lugaresi had seen a problem coming—if his patient died during *Ferragosto*, the long summer break, where would he find a pathologist to take out the brain? So Lugaresi arranged to pay one out of his pocket to be on call twenty-four hours a day. "It wasn't from Christian compassion," he says. "We knew we had some-thing. We didn't want to lose the brain." Accordingly, even though Sil-vano died just before *Ferragosto*, a pathologist arrived within hours to remove his brain, immerse it in formalin, and ship it to Pierluigi Gam-betti, a former student of Lugaresi's, who now ran a neuropathology lab at Case Western Reserve University in Cleveland. ("Why did Gambetti go to Cleveland?" Lugaresi said to me one day, looking at the lovely foothills of the Apennines outside his office. "Boh.") The rest of Silvano's body was returned to his hometown, where a funeral was held in the graveyard that had seen so much of his family's misery.

Lugaresi had never seen brain waves like Silvano's: for one thing, deep sleep was totally absent. For another, every once in a while, Silvano would go directly from a waking state into a version of REM sleep without passing through the intermediate steps—alpha to theta to sleep spindle to delta waves. And, even odder, Silvano's REM left him free to move—he could tie his tie or salute the queen—whereas normal REM sleep was characterized by total paralysis.

Even without EEGs, neurologists had learned a certain amount about sleep. Walter Rudolf Hess, who won the Nobel Prize in 1949 for his work, showed that inserting an electrode into the hippocampus of a cat would make it fall asleep. Around the same time came the great encephalitis lethargica outbreak after World War I. Millions caught the mysterious disease and were reduced either to somnolent inertia or ceaseless hyperactivity. The epidemic gave the great Austrian neurologist Constantin Von Economo an endless supply of brains to examine. What he found confirmed and extended Hess's experiments: in people who could not sleep, one part of the hypothalamus was damaged; in people who could not wake up, another part was. A later study at Pisa added a section of the brain stem to the list of structures in the brain that controlled sleep.

So, in Cleveland, Gambetti, following Elio Lugaresi's instructions, now looked carefully at Silvano's hypothalamus and his brain stem. He sectioned them with exquisite care. Strangely, the hypothalamus and the brain stem—indeed, all the brain tissue—looked healthy—except for gaps and star-shaped clusters (astrocytes) in the thalamus. In fact, the disease had destroyed 90 percent of some parts of that organ.

The finding intrigued both Gambetti and Lugaresi. The thalamus is a part of the brain that scientists don't understand well, but it appears to have a role in emotions as well as in monitoring and controlling signals that go from the hindbrain—the oldest part of the brain—to the rest of the brain and from there to the body and back. One of the thalamus's roles is as a stoplight for autonomic impulses, like temperature control, hormone release, and sweating. Neurochemicals tell the stoplight when to go from green, wakefulness, to red, sleep. But Silvano's thalamus had been eaten away to the point where no quantity of brain chemicals could change it from green to red. No wonder he had sweated uncontrollably. His body had been firing nonstop.

But why insomnia? Other than Von Economo's disease, there were a handful of conditions—most notably, delirium tremens—that caused insomnia as devastating as Silvano's, but there was no good information on what part of the brain they damaged. Yet it seemed clear that the thalamus had a key role in sleep, a role not previously understood. In fact, the Nobel laureate Hess had also done some studies connecting the thalamus to the sleep-wake cycle in cats, but subsequent researchers were not able to repeat the findings and his own more persuasive work on the hippocampus carried the day. (Damage to the thalamus would later be shown to cause the sleeplessness in delirium tremens; the doctors who kept insisting on Assunta's alcoholism were not so far off the mark.)

Ignazio, Gambetti, and Lugaresi were thrilled by their discovery. They gave the syndrome the tentative name familial hyper-somnolence. The group thought later of calling it "lethal familial insomnia," but Gambetti said, "I think 'fatal' would be better," and they all agreed. "Fatal familial insomnia" was memorable and got the disease publicity out of all proportion to the number of its sufferers. "We had a great success with the name," Gambetti remembered. "Fatal familial insomnia was much easier than familial fatal insomnia, which was probably more correct." The group published its results in 1986. But though the disease now had a name, the precise cause of the perpetually green light continued to elude researchers. What was hollowing out the thalamus?

Why was there no inflammation? Why did the disease typically strike in late middle age?

If they were to answer these questions, Lugaresi and Gambetti needed to get more information and more brains. Lisi and Ignazio set out to build a detailed family history. They re-created the family tree, which had disappeared in Padua. Lisi called relatives she barely knew to ask whether they knew of anyone who had died under odd circumstances. Ignazio had become an amateur genealogist over the years. An accomplished organist, he would go to neighboring churches and ask to see their instrument, then sneak into the parish archives with his camera to search for the family surname. In this way, they assembled a list of the victims of the disease within the family and their supposed causes. Luigi, Pietro's younger brother, had been diagnosed with encephalitis and died tied to a hospital bed in Venice in 1930. Their younger sister, Angela, died in 1948 at a mental hospital to which she had been committed for "*dispiacere,*" unhappiness or sorrow. There was Lisi's mother's cousin Maria, who had lived in Friuli and been diagnosed as a paranoid schizophrenic in 1960 at age twenty-one: she told the admitting physician she had discovered the secret of Fatima but could only reveal it to the pope, prophesied earthquakes, and complained that bugs came out of her mouth every time she spoke. The institute treated her with a combination of electroshock and insulin, which promptly killed her. At her death, the physician noted her temperature exceeded 110 degrees, the maximum reading on his thermometer.

Maria's death in turn unleashed a spate of FFI in her branch of the family: her mother, Emma; and Emma's younger sister, Irma, who was already grieving over the death of her own daughter Rita. Ignazio and Lisi were the first to associate all these deaths with a single cause. Until them, the cause of the family deaths had always been seen as a disease of exhaustion, brought on by stress or shock: Rita had seen a bloody automobile accident; a turkey had menaced Graziella.

Ignazio also found two brothers, Primo and Secondo, first cousins of Lisi's grandfather Pietro, who had both been sent to San Servolo, the mental hospital in Venice's lagoon. Primo had had fourteen children, including Giuseppe, born in 1933 in the industrial slum of Portogruaro. Theirs had been a rough life: a brother had been run over by a tractor. Giuseppe had been smart enough to realize the future for him lay elsewhere and had immigrated to Switzerland. He was physically impressive, remembered in the family as a *"uomo colossale,"* a huge man, who once killed a bull with a knife. In his mid-forties, in 1979, he developed problems walking and began to hallucinate. Like Maria, Giuseppe was diagnosed with schizophrenia, and when he died, the doctors put meningitis on his death certificate as well. But Swiss pathologists were more careful than Italian ones, and the neurologist who autopsied Giuseppe preserved some of the brain because he wasn't convinced of his own diagnosis. Ignazio was able to retrieve portions of it and send it to Gambetti to examine the thalamus. Both were disappointed when it turned out to be too decayed to make a diagnosis from.

Some members of the family simply refused to accept the news Ignazio and Lisi brought. One, a businessman whose branch of the family was free of the ailment, came to Ignazio and Lisi's house to insist that Silvano and the others had had some sort of delayed response to generations of pellagra—impossible, of course. In truth, the information that Lisi and Ignazio were dredging up was not easy for anyone to absorb. Lisi herself was frequently unable to sleep. But the search for the origins of the disease also gave her and Ignazio a shared purpose, a way to cope with what was going on around them. In 1985, Lisi's mother, Isolina, turned sixty-five, and Lisi and Ignazio were confident that she was past the age of FFI. Lisi was safe. Soon after, they conceived their daughter, Beatrice, born in 1986. (Isolina died the next year of ovarian cancer.)

When **Gambetti** and **Lugaresi** published their findings in *The New England Journal of Medicine* in 1986, they expected the medical world to be excited, but they did not count on the sharp-eyed Italian press picking up the story as well. One paper ran a picture of Lugaresi and the top of Silvano's head peeking out from under the blanket, where he had contracted into a fetal position near the end of his life. "Death comes as a liberation," the paper's correspondent assured readers. "Help Me, We Are Dying of Insomnia," ran the headline on the front page of another. Articles spoke of a century-old family curse and of Silvano's "interminable agony." One paper said another family member was about to die, while another quoted Lugaresi as saying that with Silvano the curse had ended; the family was extinct. "Let's hope that isn't just a pious lie," the savvy journalist concluded. The articles ran at the same time as a new and confusing ailment was afflicting the cows of Britain, turning that nation's usually placid meadows into the stuff of Italian nightly news. There was no small amount of delight in watching the snooty British cope with their epidemic—it had happened often enough the other way around. When the mad cow scare reached Italy, as Lisi remembers, youngsters from their neighborhood came by mooing at her door.

In all this time, the family had still never heard of prions, and prion researchers had still never heard of the family: all that was known in the 1980s about FFI was that it was a genetic disease that destroyed the thalamus, but within a few years the two worlds, the world of FFI and the world of prions, would finally come together and real progress would be made in understanding the condition.

A few years after Beatrice's birth, a cousin of Lisi's named Lucia called Ignazio and told him that her sister was behaving oddly. Teresa was bumping into furniture as she walked around the house; she was also sweating profusely. Lucia added that her father and uncle had both died of a similar disease in the late 1970s; she knew her sister's condition was not leukoencephalitis, as the doctors claimed, and she was tired of the denial that characterized her family's approach to their disease. This was the first time her branch and Lisi's had ever been in contact.

At Ignazio's urging, Lucia took Teresa to Bologna. Of all the deaths the clinicians witnessed, hers may have been the saddest: she was just thirty-six years old and had two little boys. In her first videotaped moments at the clinic, she seems cheerful, dressed in a scarlet sweater, with a soft face and full lips. Even a few months later, when her head inclines forward in a vain attempt to sleep, if a researcher taps her, she snaps to and smiles. But the disease is implacable. Over time it strips away the softness of her cheeks. Enormous black circles develop around her eyes with their pinprick pupils. Like other family members, Teresa eventually fell into an exhausted quasi-coma, her face twitching continuously, and died. Soon after, an older cousin named Luigia followed the same course with the same end. In each case, Lugaresi had a pathologist ready to extract the brain and send it to Pierluigi Gambetti in Cleveland.

Examining Luigia's and Teresa's tissue, Gambetti began to see something meaningful—at the same time as Lugaresi was beginning to detect an intriguing pattern in their EEGs.

The key was that both had a slower form of FFI than Assunta, Pierina, and Silvano had had—this slower form took several years to run its course instead of just one; so it left more extensive traces of its path of destruction. Like their kin, the sufferers from the "slow form" of FFI could not sleep, they acted out their dreams, and their EEGs were a bizarre assortment of speeded-up highs and super lows. Their bodies were also not obeying circadian rhythms, pumping out hormones day and night. There were two important clinical differences, though, between their FFI and the fast kind. First, there was a pattern of multiple spikes on their EEGs that looked to Lugaresi intriguingly similar to the brain waves of patients suffering from Creutzfeldt-Jakob disease. And when Gambetti looked at their brains, in addition to holes in the thalamus, he saw spongy areas elsewhere in the brain. To his knowledge, these patches were characteristic of only two hereditary neurological diseases, CJD and GSS.

Gambetti and Lugaresi came to the same conclusion along parallel tracks: FFI was another inherited prion disease. To test this hypothesis, they needed Stanley Prusiner's help. In the prion world, it is better to get along with Prusiner than not, and fortunately Gambetti did. "I knew Prusiner before he was Prusiner," Gambetti says, and Prusiner appreciated this. He gave Gambetti antibodies to help him test for the presence of prions in his FFI tissues; Gambetti found that, indeed, not just in Teresa's and Luigia's cases but in all the other cases of FFI—fast and slow—the tissue of the sufferer was full of malignant prions. Those malignant prions were hollowing out the thalamus and causing the disease's symptoms. (Subsequent experiments showed that mice whose prion genes had been removed displayed an intriguing tendency toward insomnia, suggesting that it might be the absence of normally formed prions rather than the destruction of the thalamus that gave the disease its most noteworthy symptom. This interpretation was also given support when Prusiner's lab discovered in 1997 that fatal insomnia could occur sporadically, just as CJD can.)

Gambetti knew Prusiner, in turn, had a problem that he could help with—he was at an impasse in an important experiment in his ongoing attempt to convince skeptics that prions caused infection without the help of hidden nucleic acids. One hurdle the theory faced was to show how prions could cause different diseases in different animals. Establishing this ability was important because some researchers believed that the target animal rather than the donor determined the symptoms in prion diseases, which suggested in turn that the prion wasn't itself infectious but rather provoked a latent infection in the target animal.

Prusiner had been working to prove these skeptics wrong. When he injected tissue from a CJD victim into mice with human prion genes, the mice got CJD: they lost coordination and eventually collapsed. But when he shot tissue from a GSS victim into mice, they didn't get sick. FFI represented a new prion disease he could use in his experiment, and Gambetti had all the tissue. In the mid-1990s, Gambetti sent FFI specimens to San Francisco to help his colleague out.

With FFI, Prusiner got the response he wanted: the CJD prion caused loss of coordination and death in mice, while the FFI prions caused sleeplessness as well as loss of coordination. Prusiner was even able to purify the FFI prions and demonstrate that their weight differed from CJD or GSS prions, suggesting that the difference among prion diseases came out of the physical difference in the arrangement of a given prion's atoms. Thanks to the experiment, Prusiner had successfully shown that different strains of prions caused specific, distinct diseases—a key feature in the definition of an infectious agent. He was one giant step closer to proving that prions and prions alone were responsible for infection.

In 1997, a year after FFI helped to pin down the mystery of prion strains, the Karolinska Institute awarded Prusiner the Nobel Prize in physiology or medicine for "a new biological principle of infection." "There are still people who don't believe that a protein can cause these diseases, but we believed it," one member of the institute told *The New York Times.* "From our point of view there is no doubt." The presentation speech emphasized Prusiner's courage, noting the "uneven battle" he had fought against "overwhelming opposition." Prusiner's detractors—those who thought he'd stolen their credit and those who thought there was no credit to steal—were horrified.

Among them was Carleton Gajdusek, who heard about Prusiner's honor from a jail cell. His refusal to conform had cost him. The Anga boy who had come to Dulles Airport in 1963, barefoot and with a bone through his nose, had been only the first. Fifty-six Micronesian and Melanesian preteens had lived with Gajdusek over the years. He had had to move to a larger house to accommodate them all. His ambition for them, he wrote in his journal, was to give them "an eye opening acquaintance with the culture of the West sufficient that they may avoid falling victims to it." Their parents had begged "Docta America" to take their kids and show them the gifts of the West: education, money, medical care. What exactly had Gajdusek wanted with all these kids? Visitors to his unconventional household took what they saw at face value: Gajd was Peter Pan; the Micronesians were his imported Lost Boys.

The FBI turned its attention to the question of whether something inappropriate was going on in Gajdusek's house in the mid-1990s, when a dissatisfied member of Gajdusek's lab—Gajdusek had turned down one of his proposals—tipped them off to the existence of his diaries. The researcher had read some of them while looking after the house of a friend of Gajdusek's whom Gajdusek had sent a set as backup. The FBI was interested in the hints the diaries gave of pedophilia. Gajdusek was a personage, a prestige target. "This case is going to put us on the map" was how one participant described the excitement investigators felt at tracking the Nobel laureate. Federal agents found one of Gajdusek's Micronesian adoptees named John Clayton Harongsemal, who said he had been molested and would cooperate. They taped Gajdusek acknowledging on the phone to Clay that they had engaged in *sir-sir,* a Micronesian term for mutual masturbation. "Gajdusek just started rambling and we had him," the investigator remembered. As the tape shows, Gajdusek felt he had been doing Clay a favor. He believed that what he'd seen on his travels showed that early homosexual behavior was useful for a successful heterosexual life. This was a minority point of view and a self-serving one at that. "I don't care about—about Papua New Guinea's culture. I'm trying to say that what you did is wrong," Clay told Gajdusek with anguish. But Gajdusek didn't see it that way—and never will.

The accusation put much of Gajdusek's previous life and work in question. Had he missed the true cause of kuru because he was so entranced with the Anga and their "semen eating"? Had all his work in New Guinea been motivated by a desire to have access to preteens? One man allegedly molested by Gajdusek in New Guinea, the adopted son of one of his friends, told a Maryland criminal investigator that Gajdusek had used his medical expertise to try to seduce him. He had diagnosed an adhesion of the foreskin and then attempted to fellate the boy.

Those who were with Gajdusek during the kuru explorations don't accept the suggestion that pedophiliac impulses were what drove him. "I have a fair experience of the seamy side of things and if he was running a bloody whorehouse I think I would have known," said Jack Baker, the Papua New Guinea patrol officer who, with his dog Kuru, accompanied Gajdusek on many of his treks through the Highlands. Under intense questioning from Clay during the taped phone call, Gajdusek acknowledged that he "touched a couple of kids" but then could name only one. None of the boys other than Clay who had spent time in Gajdusek's house said he molested them. The FBI did not believe their denials, assuming, as one agent said, that the kids "didn't want to give up the gravy train and go back to living in grass huts, wearing sarongs, and hearing about America over the transistor radio."

In February 1997, a Maryland court sentenced Gajdusek to eighteen months in county jail with the understanding that he would only have to serve less than a year. Prominent people—everyone from Linus Pauling to the novelist Arthur C. Clarke—petitioned the judge for clemency; conspicuously absent from this group was Stanley Prusiner. Now in jail, hearing the news that Prusiner had won a Nobel Prize for a "new biological principle of infection," Gajdusek was outraged. Wasn't that what he'd won *his* Nobel Prize for?

In his journal he attacked the new laureate: "I never heard a word of original thought from you nor read such ideas in anything you authored for which I did not recognize immediately its source, which you always went out of your way to obscure. You a heretic? You a martyr? You a defender of unacceptable ideas? Bullshit!! You shrewdly jumped onto a bandwagon of creative ideas and experimental work and shrewdly got onto the winning cart, proclaiming outrageously in press and media it was yours! I respect you less and less as your despicable game succeeds and you bask in your coveted fame." Sitting in jail, Gajdusek vowed never to use the word "prion."

PART III

NATURE PUSHES BACK

CHAPTER 10

APOCALYPSE COW BRITAIN, *1986*

One is a novelty. Two is a coincidence. Three is a problem.

——MARTIN JEFFREY, pathologist, Central
Veterinary Laboratory, co-discoverer of BSE

Thanks in large part to Gajdusek and Prusiner, by the mid-1980s, prion research was prestigious. Top postdocs wanted to work in the field, where not long before they would have considered studying the scrapie disease family a dead end, assuming they'd even heard of it. Prusiner and Gajdusek spent a lot of time separately spreading their gospel. They were regulars at international conferences on Alzheimer's and other neurodegenerative diseases, where they would introduce colleagues to the mystery of a disease that could be inherited, sporadic, and infectious and hint at how it might shed light on some of medicine's enduring mysteries. Listening researchers were left wondering whether the diseases they'd devoted their lives to were half so interesting.

A working theory of prion disease was falling in place: prions were ordinary proteins, created by ordinary genes, that somehow got tangled up and caused other proteins to get tangled up in turn. Prion scientists thought they had a pretty good idea of how this tangling took place on the cellular and molecular level. There was, though, nearly total uncertainty about how prion diseases actually spread in nature—but, then, except for a bunch of sheep, a few old women in New Guinea, and a handful of families like the Italian one afflicted with a genetic form of prion disease, almost no one suffered from one.

What prion researchers lacked was a significant real-life application for their work, one that would promote it from curiosity to medical necessity and pay them back in money and prestige for all the time and effort they had expended unraveling its secrets. That opportunity came in the late 1980s when a prion plague struck Britain's cattle herds and brought with it the largest public food scare of the century. The outbreak has infected at least 800,000 cattle and 160 humans to date. At first it appeared that bovine spongiform encephalopathy (informally called mad cow disease) would be the perfect opportunity for prion researchers to show their stuff, but it quickly turned out to be the opposite. In the end, the mad cow outbreak proved just how little anyone knew about prions.

In part, the insularity and insecurity of the British were responsible for this missed opportunity. The nation's politicians and scientists kept American experts like Prusiner and Gajdusek at arm's length, refusing to share data and tissue with them. Gajdusek was not taken seriously. He represented the amateurish tradition the British themselves were trying to leave behind. The antipathy for Prusiner ran far deeper and was more personal: the British hated his arrogance. They had done the original work on scrapie when the only tools available were a mouse, a syringe, and a microscope, and they weren't going to let a high-tech, press-loving chemist who knew nothing of veterinary science steal the show.

This refusal to consult with the Americans cost the British. Their scientists never caught up with the mad cow outbreak: during the decade in which it played out, each day brought them a new surprise. Prusiner, for instance, could have helped them quickly establish which parts of a cow were most dangerous to eat with his superb prion antibodies, but he was ignored. In 1990, as mad cow teetered on the edge of becoming a human epidemic, Prime Minister Margaret Thatcher reminded the British electorate that they had the best scientists working on the problem. In fact they did not. And if they had known how untrue the Iron Lady's words were, they would have given up their Cornish pasties and beefburgers a lot sooner.

The mad cow story is not a simple one. It can even be seen as the greatest epidemiological triumph in a century. But while it's true that British government scientists located the source of the mad cow infection quickly, roughly eight years passed after that discovery before an effective barrier was set up to protect humans from mad cow. It's as if John Snow had successfully traced cholera to the Broad Street pump only to have the government tell Londoners to go on drawing their water from it while committee after committee studied the problem. During the eight years between the discovery and the effective prevention of BSE, about 200,000 infected cows and between 600,000 and 1.6 million cows with preclinical indications of BSE went into the food chain and from there to Britain's supermarkets.

It can be estimated, based on a European Union scientific committee's work, that the English ate as many as 640 billion doses of BSE during the crisis as a whole. As it happens, BSE crosses from cow to human only with difficulty, but this fact wasn't anything the British government knew. They underestimated the initial threat, ignored the unique nature of the disease agent—England's chief epidemiologist wasn't a believer in prions—and allowed bureaucracy and cattle industry profits to trump speed and openness. When in doubt, they formed a committee. The one thing they had on their side was luck. Fortunately, prions aren't as infectious as, say, the flu. If they were, only long-time vegetarians would be alive in England today.

Seen in retrospect, it seems likely that as early as the late 1970s something out of the ordinary was happening on Britain's farms. In milking parlors, dairy cows, normally the gentlest of animals, were kicking herdsmen. In the field, the cows would tremble, walk clumsily and fall down. Sometimes they did not get up, or, if they did, they could barely stand, shifting their weight back and forth to balance. Soon after, they would collapse and die.

A cow is not a sheep or a pig—it is a valuable animal. When a cow dies, it isn't just picked up by the hunt club for the hounds: the farmer wants to know what happened. All the same, cows are also not humans, and the farmer needs to make money to keep farming, which means he has to keep his vet bills down. All modern veterinary medicine is done within this framework, which in practical terms translates into "look, but don't spend too much time looking."

When English vets first saw a few cows falling down, they diagnosed a mineral or organic imbalance. Cows suffer from several such problems, the most frequent being magnesium deficiency. A magnesium-deficient cow will shiver and convulse; it may appear excited or agitated. It may collapse. A cow that seems fine in the afternoon may be dead by nightfall. The technical name for the syndrome is hypomagnesemia, but the phrase that farmers use is "grass staggers," or just "staggers," because of the way the cow walks when it is getting sick.

Until the late nineteenth century, "staggers" was another name for scrapie. There was still a lot of scrapie in Britain in the 1980s, but it was a chronic problem with no cure and no human health implications, and so farmers didn't much worry about it. If they had, they might have noticed the similarities between scrapie sheep and these sick cows. The sick cows were alert and anxious, as if slightly overwhelmed by their situation. Sick cows licked themselves neurotically, much as sheep scraped themselves relentlessly against walls and posts. The sick cow held her head in an uncomfortable upright way, so marked that an experienced farmer could pick an afflicted cow out of a herd just by sight. The look was similar to the *"tête haute"* and *"regarde fixe"* that the French veterinarian Roche-Lubin noticed in infected sheep in the middle of the nineteenth century. If you stroked a cow with the staggers on its back you would elicit the same smacking, nibbling response that scrapie-affected sheep gave when scratched.

When English cows began falling ill in the late 1970s, there was another strong economic motive for farmers not to spend too much time and money on the diagnosis. If a sick cow died on the farm, you couldn't sell it into the human food chain. So when a cow with staggers didn't respond to treatment, the farmer shipped it off quickly to the slaughterhouse, where it fetched a fine price and made perfectly good eating—indeed, some food manufacturers actually preferred the lean carcasses of scrapie sheep, claiming it made for better lamb pies.

The problem of the staggering cows percolated over the years—a few cows in Surrey, a few in Hertfordshire. In the early 1980s it began to intensify, and the more interested vets began to notice it. One of them, Raymond Williams, was thirty-four years old when he saw a sick cow in the fall of 1983 on a farm in Wiltshire in southern England. The cow was anxious, kept to itself along the edges of the walk from the milking parlor to the examination pen, and was losing weight even though she ate normally. It was sometimes too aggressive to be milked.

The owner of the farm was a man whose family had once owned the entire valley in which he lived, the principal village of which, Castle Combe, had been the site of the 1966 movie *Doctor Doolittle*. But this farmer was no romantic animal lover; he used a computerized system to monitor his 250-cow herd. His program showed how to maximize milk production by adjusting the content of feed. The sick cow was eventually slaughtered and shipped to market.

In the months that followed, two more cows got sick on the same farm. Then a fourth cow fell ill. Raymond Williams took the unusual step of slaughtering the cow himself, sawing off its head, and taking out some of the brain. He also removed the liver and the abomasum, the one of the cow's four stomachs that absorbs nutrients and where toxins generally wind up. He sent the stomach to a government veterinary lab in Gloucester and the liver and brain to researchers at the Glasgow University veterinary school, where he'd trained. The findings that came back were "nonspecific." One pathologist speculated that the cow had grazed near a discarded car battery: leaking lead could cause a pathology similar to the one he had observed.

Then a fifth cow got sick. At Williams's suggestion, the farmer shipped the cow live to the University of Bristol. He added one request: if it was put down and given a postmortem, the farmer didn't want it hacked up so badly that it couldn't be sold for human consumption. At Bristol, veterinarians ran a lot of tests and, during this time, believed the cow was recovering. Their best guess was that an electrical fault in the milking parlor was causing the excitability and perhaps the declining milk production. The farmer was taking no chances. He ordered the cow slaughtered, and it too went into the food chain. The government vet expressed the hope that whatever had been going on was now over. But about a hundred miles away, in Sussex, a veterinarian named David Bee, unaware of what was going on near Castle Combe, was seeing similar cases. He, too, was sending cows for autopsy and getting back negative results. Eventually he sent a live cow to a government-run veterinary investigative center. The cow had been shaking and falling. At the VIC, government vets euthanized the cow, mounted brain tissue on slides, and forwarded them to the government's Central Veterinary Laboratory on the southwest edge of London.

A pathologist named Carol Richardson drew the random assignment to examine the tissue from the cow in September 1985. Richardson was not a star, even in the low-key world of veterinary pathology, but as it happened, she was very curious about scrapie. As a student in the 1970s, she had had a mentor who had delighted her with its mysteries. Under a microscope, he had shown her the holes that riddled the brain and described the controversy surrounding the cause, how the infectious agent had never been isolated. When Richardson saw the same pattern of holes in the brain in the cow that her teacher had long ago shown her in sheep, she immediately understood what she was seeing. "The hairs on the back of my head went all tingly," she remembered. "I thought, This is scrapie in a cow."

With eagerness, Richardson walked the slides down the hall to have a colleague confirm her observation. That confirmation never came. Her colleague, Gerald Wells, looked at the slides and read her report and doubted her findings. He considered how many things cause holes in a cow's brain and gave the report back to Richardson recommending a diagnosis of fungal toxin. She acquiesced even without agreeing and sent a letter back to David Bee, the veterinarian, with Wells's conclusions. Fungal toxin was a dead-end diagnosis, the veterinary equivalent of "Boh." Bee was disappointed, but the syndrome disappeared from his client's farm. He moved on, just as Raymond Williams had.

Six more months passed. Now another veterinarian, Colin Whitaker, was running into odd cows on a farm in Kent. The farm was large, a piece of the holdings that had belonged to Lord Plurenden, a refugee from the Nazis who had become the powerful chairman of the British Agricultural Export Council. Plurenden had died in 1978, but his business interests lived on. The farm's cows were pedigreed, top producers; they won prizes in local competitions.

Whitaker's sick cows were particularly aggressive. They charged when challenged and turned to try to bite if forced into the milking press. "It was quite dangerous," Whitaker remembered—and confusing. Whitaker called in the local government veterinary officer, who sent two brains to the government pathology laboratory, where Gerald Wells, the man who had overruled Richardson's diagnosis of bovine scrapie in David Bee's cow, received them. Wells and Whitaker were friends, former college roommates. Whitaker explained what he had seen, and Wells took the tissue, had it examined under an electron microscope, considered the history his college roommate gave him, and had no doubt that he was looking at a case of scrapie in a cow. He was thrilled by the opportunity to make medical history. He says he had no memory of the report Richardson showed him the year before. He went down the hall to share his discovery with another colleague, Martin Jeffrey.

As it happened, Jeffrey had recently been called in by a zoo in Hampshire to examine tissue from a nyala—an antelope-like animal in the bovine family that had died mysteriously. The nyala's brain was full of holes. "I have something interesting to show you," Wells told Jeffrey. And Jeffrey answered: "I have something interesting to show you, too." Then they went down the hall to tell their boss, Raymond Bradley, the head of the pathology department, the remarkable news that scrapie appeared to have jumped species. They had discovered a new disease, and not just a new disease but one with important economic ramifications. They were, Wells remembers, very excited. This was what they had become pathologists to do.

Bradley shared their excitement but also felt anxiety: for British beef eaters. While scrapie had never crossed to humans, scrapie in cows might. You could not assume anything with such a poorly understood disease. He sent off a memo—he loved memos, writing them by hand when the women in the typing pool were busy—to that effect to his superior, a man named Howard Rees, the chief veterinary officer.

Rees did not thrill to the mystery of what was going on. "My first thought was of the industry," he remembered. America had banned the import of British sheep in the 1950s and consumption of sheep and lamb from scrapie-infected flocks in 1976, a decision that cost Britain money every year. For this reason, Rees tried to keep the news from getting out until his agency could prove or disprove a link to scrapie. Needless to say, that standard of proof would have to be quite high.

Conferring regularly with his higher-ups in the Ministry of Agriculture, Fisheries and Food, Rees decided to confine within MAFF what little information his veterinarians had. He knew there were brighter minds on scrapie at universities and research institutes in Britain and abroad who could help—who would *love* to help—but he wasn't going to give them a chance.

Since most of the veterinarians who knew about the problem worked for Rees, for a time he was able to keep a lid on the news. A paper Gerald Wells was working on about the first cases he had seen was cut in half on Rees's order, a line drawn just above where the word "scrapie" first appeared. A paper Jeffrey wanted to publish on the nyala was held back and a presentation by the veterinarian Colin Whitaker, who had seen the cases on Lord Plurenden's farm, was censored. Whitaker had prepared a list of seventeen possible causes for the new condition. Number seventeen read "A New Scrapie-like Syndrome[?]." When MAFF was done, the word "scrapie-like" had disappeared. "It was just 'A New' and then a great big black blob, then 'Syndrome,' " Whitaker remembered, still angry.

By May 1987, MAFF counted nineteen confirmed or suspected cases of the new cow disease. What was the disease and where did it come from? The man the agency chose to look into the question was an epidemiologist named John Wilesmith. His specialty was tuberculosis in badgers—he knew next to nothing about scrapie—but MAFF liked him because as an employee of the agency he could be controlled.

A new disease outbreak is essentially a logical puzzle. The first question you ask is, What do all the cases have in common? The second is whether anything was done to the sick that wasn't also done to the well. The intersection point of these two questions is the source of the problem. In theory, it's not that complicated.

But in the case of this new disease, several factors made it harder.

First, scrapie was poorly understood. Second, the disease was still an official secret. Third, the lives of cows are heavy with human intervention. They are fed, sprayed, impregnated, milked, housed, and pastured by people, and there are differences in these agricultural practices from region to region—say, from Scotland to Somerset. In addition, farmers keep poor records, and they tell stories that are sometimes more folklore than fact. Amateur curers crisscross England selling home remedies the contents of which farmers only half understand. "Half a vet's time is spent checking what's on the farmer's shelf," Wilesmith said.

Wilesmith began visiting farms in June 1987 with local veterinarians like David Bee and Colin Whitaker in tow. His manner was deliberately pleasant and unthreatening—he knew it was unsettling enough to a farmer for a placid cow he'd known its whole life to turn mad in front of his eyes without having a government vet officer poke around asking about it afterward. At the time it was still legal to send a sick cow to the slaughterhouse so long as it could walk, but you did not have to be brilliant to see that if MAFF had taken the trouble to send an epidemiologist to your farm, that situation might quickly change. Wilesmith knew the first trick would be to get farmers to trust him with what they had seen.

Wilesmith's first suspicion was that scrapie had contaminated a vaccine for cows. The fact that the outbreak appeared to have started at a number of places almost at the same time argued for multiple simultaneous infections, and experience told Wilesmith that there was no more likely cause for them than an injection. He was also thinking of the accidental scrapie outbreak that the veterinarian W. S. Gordon started in Scotland in the 1930s, when he was trying to perfect his vaccine against louping-ill. But Wilesmith's interviews with farmers did not turn up an injected medicine all the cows had in common.

He then moved on to insecticides. Farmers exposed British cows to a remarkable number of chemicals—Ridect for flies and Valbazen,

Ivomec, and Paratect for worms. They poured Tiguvon, essentially a highly toxic nerve gas, on the cows' backs to protect against warble fly. Wilesmith grew most interested in a chemical called a pyrethroid, an artificial version of a chrysanthemum derivative that farmers soaked cows' ear tags in to keep away flies. Pyrethroids were most often used in the south of England, where most of the flies were, and most of the cases of this new scrapie-like illness in cows were occurring. But events at the Central Veterinary Laboratory, over the previous seven months of observing cow brains under a microscope, overtook this line of inquiry. Pathologists there had discovered that, besides having holes in them, the cows' brains contained small amyloid protein plaques: clumps of dead brain protein. They did not see how pyrethroids could produce the plaques, which were caused in the animal world only by scrapie.

In the meantime, Colin Whitaker, the veterinarian who had seen the cases at Lord Plurenden's farm, gave his presentation, the one MAFF had censored, at a conference of British cattle veterinarians. He talked about the aggressive, trembling cows he had seen in Kent. Despite the editing he had undergone, his audience knew what they were hearing. David Bee, the veterinarian who had seen even earlier cases, happened to be there. He popped up afterward. "I've seen that," he said, to Whitaker's irritation. "Sounds like scrapie in a cow," other vets commented. In the months that followed, various farm journals wrote up the nameless disease, followed by *The Daily Telegraph,* the first national daily to do so, which in October 1987 gave the news that "a mystery brain disease is killing Britain's dairy cows, and vets have no cure."

MAFF gave the disease an official name, bovine spongiform encephalopathy, for the opposite reason Stanley Prusiner had called transmissible viral spongiform encephalopathies "prion diseases"— the ministry wanted the term forgotten as quickly as possible. Bovine spongiform encephalopathy was a disease that, *The Economist* complained, "twists the tongues of vets and wrecks the brains of cows." The name hardly did justice to BSE's spectacular symptoms: cows kicking their handlers, charging herdsmen on their knees, head-butting. Newspapers assayed several adjectives to capture what was going on—there were "nutty" cows, then "silly" ones, "bloody mad" cows, and then, finally, the *Sunday Telegraph* wrote of the "incurable 'mad cow disease' which riddled the brain with holes and drove docile animals berserk." MAFF hated the name, but it stuck.

Wilesmith was working hard now to solve the mystery but his superiors were mired in MAFF's inherent conflict of interest between protecting Britain's agriculture business and the safety of its food supply.

At the same time, the pathologists back at the Central Veterinary Laboratory were having their own problems: they could not keep up with the brains pouring in for autopsy. Their counterparts at a research facility in Edinburgh that had long specialized in scrapie said they could confirm BSE in a cow in a day using a version of the antibody test that Prusiner and other labs had developed. The Americans too stood ready to help. But the CVL preferred to keep slicing brains, staining the tissue and putting it on slides—a process that could take weeks—to look for the telltale holes and amyloid plaques. For them, it was as if the previous ten years of prion research had never taken place.

By November 1987, there were thirty-two confirmed cases of BSE and ninety-six suspected ones, spread out over more than fifty farms. The majority of farms had a single case. One farm, though, had eleven. Most farmers were still quietly shipping their affected cattle to market. By now, Wilesmith had considered and ruled out chemical, environmental, and genetic causes. That left food as a suspect, but like all epidemiologists, Wilesmith resisted the idea of food-borne infections, because digestive acids do an excellent job of sterilizing the stomach's contents. It's hard to get sick from something you eat. But in the feed records of farmers, Wilesmith kept noticing, the words "cake in parlour" appeared over and over like a sinister nursery rhyme.

The "cake," or high-protein concentrate, was usually given during milking, that is, "in parlour," because then the cow was alone and could be given a supplement tailored to her needs. Cows liked cake—it was sweetened with molasses—and they understood it as a reward for being cooperative during milking.

One important source of protein in cake was meat from other farm animals, specifically farm animals that could not be sold into the human food supply because they had died in the field. Jobbers would come and cart away "down" and dead stock and sell it to renderers. The renderers boiled the dead animals and then treated the carcasses chemically and shipped the results to feed companies, who packaged it and sold it to farmers. It was possible, if unlikely, Wilesmith thought, that some unusually tough infectious agent could survive such a journey.

Wilesmith learned several other facts that made the cake theory more attractive. Many of the sick cows were very young, which meant they had been infected just after birth. He also noticed that beef cattle herds did not suffer as many cases of BSE as dairy herds, nor were cows born to dairy herds and sent shortly after to beef herds much afflicted. Wilesmith asked himself what was happening in dairy herds that wasn't also happening in beef herds. It turned out that beef herd calves were allowed to suckle, while dairy calves were taken right from their mothers and put on concentrate because the farmers wanted the mother's milk. They did not want the calf drinking up their profits.

In January 1988, Wilesmith received a phone call from a veterinary official that strengthened the case for cake as the cause of BSE. The Marwell Zoo in Hampshire had just lost another antelope-like animal, a gemsbok, to a strange disease. This was the same zoo where the nyala had died in 1986. When an autopsy confirmed that the gemsbok suffered from a spongiform encephalopathy, Wilesmith asked its keepers the same question he was asking all the farmers: what had changed recently in the gemsbok's life? The answer was its food—the company that manufactured antelope feed pellets had replaced soy protein with meat protein for a year to lower its costs.

By now, Wilesmith was zeroing in on cake, which was also known as meat and bone meal. As he grew more certain, he asked the feed and rendering companies whether they were doing anything new with their meat processing, anything in the last five years, which was the time frame he had established for the outbreak. They told him they were using more sheep parts, especially more sheep brains. They had also lowered the temperature at which they were processing their meat and bone meal and they had stopped treating the meal with certain denaturing chemicals. Any or all of these changes might permit an agent that hadn't previously been able to survive to get into cattle feed, Wilesmith reasoned. Once he had this information, by early 1988, he felt confident enough to write up his hypothesis, that infectious scrapie particles from sheep were surviving the rendering process and infecting dairy cows through their feed, and to make his report to his bosses at MAFF.

Wilesmith had taken a complex riddle and returned with a good solution. He had done it all with minimal resources. MAFF now had a mechanism and a cause. Mad cow came from scrapie, which was a great relief for Britain's beef industry, since everyone knew eating scrapie-infected sheep did not make you sick. MAFF assumed BSE would prove similarly benign to beef eaters—no doubt there was self-interest involved—and nearly all the world's scrapie experts concurred, including Stanley Prusiner.

But the news also carried Britain's epidemiologists and veterinarians into unfamiliar waters: none of them had any idea how to predict the shape of a scrapie outbreak, how long it would last, how to mini-mize it, or whether all those stories about how scrapie was almost im-possible to get rid of would prove true for cows with scrapie too. Had Wilesmith traced BSE to a conventional virus, none of these would have been question marks. But a lot of uncertainty lay ahead. All the same, MAFF set about fixing the problem John Wilesmith had solved, naively confident that the hard part was done.

CHAPTER 11

OINKIES BRITAIN, *1996*

*I verily believe and to date there has been no information
to persuade me otherwise, that British beef kills.*

—ANTHONY BOWEN, father of mad cow
victim Michelle Bowen

In the eighteenth century, the Leicestershire breeder Robert
Bakewell "substituted profitable flesh for useless bone" to create the
barrel-shaped sheep that fed the new industrial masses of England.
Dairy farmers, noting Bakewell's achievements, tried to work parallel
magic on their cows, a project that gained momentum as life grew
more comfortable over time and the public's expectation of abundant
meat and milk increased.

Over the years, through aggressive breeding, farmers remade the
British cow. They standardized its color to black and white, widened
its nostrils, and strengthened its jaw. Most important, they made the

cow's body stronger to support enormous udders. Even the hindquarters were lifted higher, to give calves (and farmers) easier access to the teats.

Bakewell had tried to turn sheep into machines that "turned herbage . . . into money." English dairy farmers had the same hope for their cows, but they had better tools, the most important being access to semen from highly prized bulls all over the world and a better system for tracking champion bloodlines. The combination worked. Starting after World War II, English cows began to break milking record after milking record. Whereas a good cow in the 1940s might give a thousand gallons of milk in a year, and a champion might give two thousand gallons, by 1985, thirty-five hundred gallons was not unusual in a high-quality cow. One remarkable cow gave 159,880 gallons over her lifetime. A 1946 farm journal article summed up the results: "No breed can have started with more unsatisfactory animals than did the one that has been so greatly and wondrously improved."

But breeding was only one part of maximizing milk production. Feeding was the other part. As any nursing mother knows, milk production is a protein-intensive activity. Top-producing cows needed a special diet to do their work. Specifically, cows needed a protein that could survive the ruminants' first three stomachs so that it could be absorbed by the fourth. Only a tough protein could do this. As a 1963 farm journal article put it, "If you aren't prepared to feed for the extra yield, forget it,"

The man who first suggested that animal protein might fill the gap was Baron von Liebig—the same nineteenth-century German chemist who had disputed Pasteur's microbe theory of disease. In the mid-nineteenth century, Von Liebig, a professor at the University of Giessen in southwestern Germany, noticed that there were huge hide-tanning plants in South America discarding tons of beef because there was no way to ship them to Europe before they spoiled. He had read Malthus, and he had an idea for how to preserve some of that protein and help feed Europe's swelling working class. He manufactured a high-protein extract of beef, a concentrated cube, from the unwanted carcasses of South American cattle. The key was to extract the protein essence completely, so the cube would not grow rancid on the long journey to Europe.

Von Liebig scored a big success with his cube—faint-feeling women all over Europe began taking "Liebigs"—but a year or so after creating his meat essence for humans, he realized he had more to do. The runoff from his beef extract was going to waste, diminishing his profits. So he recovered it, added salt and what one journal of the time daintily called "refuse meat fibre," and fed it to pigs. The pigs didn't like it, but when the concentrate was flavored with something sweet, they would tolerate it. Soon farmers were feeding the concoction not just to pigs but to cows and chickens. (Horses refused it.)

Eventually, two kinds of animal protein were used in animal feed. There was "American meat meal," which was made from the parts of animals humans didn't eat, and there was "German cadaver meal," which was derived from the corpses of sick animals. Both helped livestock put on weight quickly, and both products were hits in the farm world. The possibility of food-borne infection from sick animals occurred to farmers at the time, but one 1909 scientific manual was typical in assuring readers that "superheated steam in large drums containing revolving knives" removed all infection from the meat and reduced the concoction to a safe powder.

Forcing a normally vegetarian farm animal to eat other farm animals turns it into an unwitting cannibal—it pits men, as Bakewell's critic Richard Parkinson said, "in opposition to their Creator"—but Von Liebig didn't see it that way. Instead, he considered himself a conservationist, improving on the natural cycle of birth, growth, and death. Few others saw the practice as immoral, either. On the contrary, shortly after World War II, the British government *required* that manufactured cow feed contain 5 percent animal protein—anything less would cheat the farmer. And over time cows came to need the supplement: focused breeding had turned every cow into a huge milk producer, and, like doping athletes, they needed something special to keep performing at full potential. Without it, they wouldn't just give less milk but would become infertile or too weak to graze. After a point, English farmers had no choice but to feed cake to their cows.

By the 1980s, the farmers participating in this race were not really interested in the money the extra milk would bring nor were they operating out of a desire to feed the masses: England already had too much milk and cheese, as had the rest of Europe. What motivated farmers was machismo. Dairy farmers live an odd life: they spend their days charting their cows' estrus and massaging ointment on their animals' sore udders. Theirs is a business where the jokes are about insemination orgies and cow is put up against cow for top milking honors. "Are you mixing with the best?" a 1985 advertisement for a dairy concentrate challenged the farmer. Feeding cows animal protein wasn't just about helping them realize their physical potential. It was about helping the farmer to realize his.

By the 1980s, the British farmer wanted to be a champion. A champion had a champion cow, and a champion cow had to have special protein. Not that the farmers knew that they were feeding cows the remains of other cows: they knew they were giving some sort of animal protein, and they weren't much interested in finding out more as long as it worked. All they knew was that every morning they still got up when it was dark, as their fathers and grandfathers had done, to keep their appointments in the milking parlor. Only now, their cows were kicking them when they got there.

It was now March 1988. Sir Donald Acheson, the chief medical officer of Britain, the equivalent of the U.S. surgeon general, was about to step onstage. In the tragedy of mad cow disease, this is the moment when we want to shout: "Look to the hamburgers, Sir Donald! Look to the meat pies! Look to the teenagers!" The government's response to the BSE epizootic was now fifteen months old. During this time the confident, creaky machine that was British government had ground along. MAFF had traced BSE to scrapie, transmitted by infected sheep-protein concentrate in cow feed. John Wilesmith's persuasive work had underscored the importance of the ministry's storied veterinary division and led to talk within the agency that BSE might have come along just in time to protect the vets from Margaret Thatcher's ever-present budget knife.

MAFF was determined to keep BSE a veterinary problem, for veterinarians. Its top officials had ignored warnings over the months from their own indefatigable memo-loving pathology lab head Raymond Bradley that it might be a good idea also to look at the *human* implications of the outbreak. Bradley's suggestion to undertake animal trials to see if BSE could pass to "primates (& by inference to man)" was approved, but MAFF's focus remained slaughtering all the sick cows in Britain as quickly as possible to reassure Britain's concerned export partners. The only way to do that was to require farmers to report BSE in their herds; farmers would in turn expect payment for the cows MAFF made them slaughter. The stumbling block was that MAFF didn't have the budget to pay compensation; it needed someone who had responsibility for human health to say BSE represented a danger to humans for the government to write a very large check. At the time, there were only about five hundred reported cases of BSE in cattle and none in people.

It turned out Sir Donald was in no hurry to help MAFF. He was nearing retirement and wasn't about to frighten people with off-the-cuff pronouncements. Never having heard of BSE and knowing little about scrapie, he felt he needed a committee of experts to help him decide what to do. He shared with other medical officials in England a great faith in scientific consensus.

The committee he convened, named the Southwood Working Party after the professor of zoology Sir Richard Southwood who headed it, first met in June 1988. Though there were no prion experts on the panel, they at once saw the risk in having BSE-infected cows in the food chain and, to MAFF's relief, they recommended the immediate reporting, slaughter, and destruction, with compensation, of all infected cattle. Immediately, the number of cases farmers reported shot up. They would quickly clean out the barn and then British beef would be back on top, MAFF thought.

The ministry did not expect its new policy to cause any particular anxiety among the public, but Britons were beginning to notice an inconsistency in their government's position. Why would it pay millions of pounds for a bunch of infected cows if there was no human risk? MAFF, joined by Sir Donald, had an answer ready: the government was acting out of an abundance of caution.

Meanwhile, the Southwood Working Party and the experts who advised it were learning on the job. They learned, for instance, that the BSE agent entered the animal through the mouth and then followed the digestive tract into the organs that try to filter out infections—the tonsils, the guts, and the spleen—and from there traveled into the peripheral and central nervous system, and finally arrived at the brain. They also learned that pasties, meat pies, and even some baby foods contained tissues from a lot of those organs. So the Southwood Working Party recommended banning these organs, but only from baby food. This started a chain reaction of consumer doubt: if infected cow organs were unsafe for babies, how could they be good for adults? The government then banned offal, as the organs were collectively called, in all human food but gave the industry a grace period to get it out of the feed supply. Then pet food manufacturers began to wonder if what drove cows mad might not also drive dogs, cats, and parrots mad. The feed they sold came from concentrate made of the same sick animals that had previously made up the meat and bone meal farmers used. Their trade group decided to put a similar ban in place—immediately. So for five months it was safer to be a dog than a human in Britain.

Publicly, government officials insisted that there was no risk to humans in eating BSE-infected tissue. Others in government saw the matter more truthfully: they knew MAFF and Sir Donald were relying on guesswork. No one really knew where BSE came from, how it was spread, and whether it could be passed to humans. "The last," wrote one undersecretary to the minister of agriculture, "seems to me the most worrying aspect of the problem. There is no evidence that people can be infected but we cannot say that there is no risk." Just because scrapie didn't transmit to humans, who knew whether the same was true of BSE? The next good information on that question wouldn't arrive until the primate trials proposed by Bradley yielded results two years later.

By 1990 the public had begun to catch on to how much less the government knew than it pretended. For one thing, the Southwood Working Party had predicted twenty thousand cases of BSE for the whole epizootic and the number was already nearly surpassed, with three hundred more cases every week and counting (it would peak at around thirty-seven thousand cases annually in 1992). Then came the announcement that a greater kudu, an Arabian oryx, and an eland at Marwell Zoo had joined the original nyala and gemsbok on the BSE victims list. More worrisome still was that an experiment to transmit BSE orally to mice was successful, proving that BSE could jump species through food. The point was underscored in May when a cat in Bristol was diagnosed with feline spongiform encephalopathy.

The discovery of feline spongiform encephalopathy in Max—"Mad Max," as he was quickly dubbed by the British papers—intensified the public's anxiety. In January 1990, Max's owner had noticed her pet was having trouble walking. Intriguingly, when she stroked his back, he made licking and chewing gestures, just like a sheep with scrapie. In April 1990, Max was euthanized; his brain was autopsied and found to be full of holes. Further examination confirmed a spongiform encephalopathy, a revelation that got enormous coverage in the British press. The public's trust was crumbling. Until this moment, the English had regarded the string of disturbing reports on the cow front complacently, but within a week of the discovery of Mad Max, school districts started banning British beef. Nearly a quarter of British consumers said they would no longer eat it.

British beef and its promoters fought back. The agriculture minister, John Gummer, fed his daughter a hamburger at a TV photo-op.* Officials went on tour to try to persuade English schools to put beef back on the menu. The Meat and Livestock Commission, a government-funded organization that helped promote British farm products, sponsored a contest to find the "tastiest and most innovative children's novelty meat product." (The winner was "Oinkies," a combination of sausage meat and cheddar balls.)

But the public now expected more bad news, and their suspicion was confirmed when in March 1991 a calf came down with BSE some three years after the cause of the outbreak—the feeding of bovine protein to cows—was supposed to have been outlawed. There were, as usual, various theories as to how the infection could have evaded the government's attempts to quell it. Some researchers thought the disease was being passed down from mother to daughter or picked up from contaminated land—the way scrapie was thought to be—but Wilesmith correctly traced the problem to manufacturers who were breaking the law, still putting cow or sheep protein in feed meant for cows. It turned out farmers were cheating too, using up their old feed.

---

* But four-year-old Cordelia made a face that suggested she'd rather be eating anything else—it was later reported that she found the hamburger too hot—and the moment registered in the British mind as only a failed photo-op can. (The phrase "doing a Gummer" remains in British political lexicon for such moments.)

They reasoned that if the government hadn't required a recall, how dangerous could the contaminated feed really be? And hadn't the government said over and over that the beef was safe?

Wilesmith also found that manufacturers were not cleaning out their equipment regularly. They might mill a shipment of cow protein for chicken feed, then mill a shipment of chicken protein for cow feed in the same machine, and one was contaminating the other. Tests confirmed the contamination—infected bovine protein was getting back into bovine feed.

The experts were beginning to realize how tricky prion epidemiology was, and the logistics of a truly comprehensive feed ban were so complicated that a new law banning animal protein in cow feed would not be put into effect until 1994. No law banning animal protein in all animal feed would be enacted until 1996, five long years after. In the meantime, the government contented itself with the knowledge that the outbreak had peaked, as fewer cases were showing up.

But more surprises had come out. Finally, the transmission experiments that Raymond Bradley had asked for at the beginning of the crisis were complete. In 1991, two marmosets inoculated with tissue from scrapie-infected sheep came down with scrapie. Marmosets are primates, like humans. The government tried to declare victory, because two other marmosets injected with BSE during the same experiment were healthy; BSE was clearly less infectious than scrapie. Unfortunately, less than a year later, the marmosets inoculated with BSE—the ones that had seemed fine—began to show symptoms of mad cow disease.

New research also suggested that the Southwood Working Party's recommendations had been too narrow; there was more infectious tissue in a sick cow than they had realized. So in 1994 eating intestines from calves two months old or older—the age at which the infectious particle appeared in the intestine—was banned. In 1995, the whole cow head except for cheek meat and the tongue was prohibited. Then cheek meat went. Finally, only the tongue could be eaten, provided it could be extracted without dislodging potentially infectious tissue elsewhere in the head.

The public found out things it never wanted to know about how beef got to the supermarket. It learned, for example, that slaughter-houses did not separate beef from offal in a delicate way. Abattoir workers were not modern-day Vesaliuses. Sometimes the cow was killed with a bullet, which could spray contaminated brain into the rest of the body. And workers used high-pressure hoses to blast tiny bits of meat off bone from areas of the carcass that were perilously near the infectious tissues of the spinal cord. The result, known as mechani-cally recovered meat—"more of a slurry than a recognized piece of meat," in the words of an unusually candid supermarket official—was a central component of hamburgers. In December 1995, the govern-ment prohibited mechanically recovering meat from the vertebrae of cattle older than six months.

There was only one shoe yet to drop—would mad cow cross to hu-mans? Then in January 1994, under a huge headline—"Mad Cow: The Human Link?"—a tabloid reported the case of sixteen-year-old Victo-ria Rimmer. Rimmer lay blind and mute in a hospital in Liverpool. She had fallen ill in early 1993. First she'd suffered memory loss—she could not find her way home from a party—then a "searing pain to her right arm and neck," and then her coordination failed. When she walked, her grandmother said, she looked like the "cows with BSE staggering on television." These were, said the paper, the classic symptoms of sporadic CJD, except that Rimmer was more than forty years younger than sporadic CJD sufferers. In addition, as her grand-mother pointedly told the papers, Victoria had "lived on" beefburgers.

The government responded with more banalities. "The facts are clear," Dr. Kenneth Calman, the chief medical officer who had re-placed Sir Donald Acheson, said. "Creutzfeldt Jakob disease is ex-tremely rare. Those who get it have contracted it for a variety of reasons. There is no evidence at all that eating infected meat is one of them." Prime Minister John Major, Margaret Thatcher's successor, himself wrote to the grieving mother of a young meat-pie maker who had died of CJD to remind her that "humans DO NOT get mad cow disease."

Privately, government officials were admitting their confusion. If Vicky Rimmer had sporadic CJD, she would be the youngest case in Britain in twenty-three years. Various independent researchers, tired of the government's evasions, were telling the newspapers that they had no doubt that Rimmer had been infected by beefburgers and sausages. "It is an inescapable conclusion that [BSE] has got into our food chain," said Stephen Dealler, a microbiologist in York and a frequent critic of MAFF. For two weeks Vicky's image was everywhere. A saucy-looking teenager with large dangling earrings and long straight hair combed over one eye, she dominated the tabloids. A reporter got a tour of her house and reported what she'd written on her wall calendar: "I want my life back."

What happened next in her case confused everyone. Vicky Rimmer didn't die. Doctors gave her months, maybe weeks to live, but she remained in a coma—not for a month, or a year, but year after year—through 1994, 1995, 1996, and most of 1997. During this time, her case dropped from sight.

But while she languished, other teens got sick with CJD, enough of them and in rapid enough succession that there was no possibility of a coincidence. The government knew that its line had become ludicrous. On March 20, 1996, Stephen Dorrell, the health secretary, stood up in Parliament to announce the news that had already appeared as a tentative conclusion in scientific journals and as rumor in newspapers for the previous two years: British beef was killing British teenagers. The first confirmed death was that of Stephen Churchill, a nineteen-year-old student from Wiltshire, who died in May 1995. Back in 1989, at the Southwood Working Party's suggestion, the government had set up a surveillance unit in Edinburgh to watch for any evidence that BSE had crossed to humans. One worry had been that if BSE passed to humans, how would anyone know it? How would you recognize something you had never seen? It turned out to be easy: Churchill and the nine other teenagers who had gotten sick had spectacular amyloid plaques in their brains, chunks of dead protein almost visible to the naked eye. If sporadic CJD was a whisper, BSE-caused prion disease was a shout. The investigators sat open-mouthed looking at slides whose damage, they feared, portended the most severe epidemic in modern British history. Noting the similarity in the pathology to sporadic and genetic CJD, they called the disease new variant CJD.

Events had humiliatingly, decisively, swung out of the control of the British government. Europe banned British beef. (John Major expressed his "astonishment" at the decision.) The bottom dropped out of beef sales in England. Supermarkets canceled their orders, livestock dealers stopped buying cattle, and farmers got stuck with a lot of cows that might or might not be safe to eat. A farmer's magazine ran a cartoon, entitled "Apocalypse Cow!," of a cow carrying a sign with the words "The End Is Nigh."

It almost was. The public wanted the slaughter of Britain's entire eleven-million-cow herd. The government resisted, still worried about cost. In the end, it decided to order the slaughter of all cattle older than thirty months, basing its decision on data showing that it took that long for the amount of prion in tissue of infected cows to become dangerous (this data would later be refuted). The government killed 3.3 million older cattle whose condition was unknown between 1996 and 1999, at a cost of billions of pounds. "The housewife wants confidence in beef," one beef processor explained in a House of Commons report. "She will get confidence in beef."

The housewife was not so easy to assuage. Just as no one had known what would happen to cattle, now no one knew what would happen to humans. Was everyone who ate meat, even once, going to die? Were only a handful? Newspapers floated scenarios reminiscent of kuru in which at the turn of the millennium a half million people a year were dying and Great Britain was quarantined. The chairman of the expert committee that had replaced the Southwood Working Party said he could not "rule out 500,000 cases," and in 1999, Britain's chief medical officer, Liam Donaldson, the replacement for Sir Donald's replacement, gave an estimate of "from under a hundred to several million" dead from BSE over the coming years.

The size of the epidemic turned out to be closer to the smaller of those two numbers. So far, one hundred and fifty Britons have died of variant Creutzfeldt-Jakob disease ("new" was gradually dropped from the disease name in the late 1990s), fewer than have died in the same period falling from ladders and a tenth as many as have drowned. There have also been cases in France, Italy, Ireland, Portugal, Spain, South Korea, and Japan that were most likely indigenous. And a twenty-five-year-old woman who spent her childhood in England died in the United States in 2004. The number of people infected with prions is far larger, though. Tests of the appendices and tonsils of otherwise healthy people in the U.K. suggest that almost four thousand Britons have the infection—although whether they will all die of mad cow, or even show symptoms, is unknown. It may be that humans can walk around with a certain amount of misformed prion in their organs and not get sick. On balance, with each passing year it appears more likely that the epidemic has peaked. Indeed, experts from Imperial College in London, who in 1997 had entertained the possibility of an epidemic of ten million, most recently classed the probable death at an upper limit of seven thousand with "95% confidence." John Collinge, a leading British prion researcher, cautions that "we shouldn't think we're out of the woods yet," but others think that he is just trying to keep the funding flowing. At the end of 2004, the British government permitted the slaughter and sale of cattle older than thirty months again, in effect declaring that, in its mind, the BSE crisis was over. The Janus aspect of the BSE epidemic—is the worst ahead or behind?—was captured in an appearance Stanley Prusiner made at an October 2005 German prion conference. Standing at the podium, seeing the seven hundred upturned faces in front of him, he pronounced the meeting the largest prion gathering to date, then added in an overheard aside that it also might well prove the largest ever.

Among the most puzzling deaths from mad cow disease was that of twenty-four-year-old Clare Tomkins. Clare lived in Kent, not far from the farm where the first cases in cows that caught MAFF's attention had appeared. She was a lively young woman with a good sense of fun. If Vicky Rimmer was England's postindustrial reality, Clare was its preindustrial fantasy. She was the classic English girl, with strawberry blond hair and cheeks that freckled in the sun. She had kept a horse and worked in a pet shop. Every week she donated part of her pay to an animal welfare fund.

Around the time of the health secretary's 1996 announcement that BSE appeared to have crossed to humans, Clare began to feel depressed. She cried uncontrollably and stopped eating. She didn't want to leave her parents' side. It was as if she had regressed to childhood.

Soon Clare began hallucinating, rocking and jerking reflexively, feeling pain in her knees and numbness in her lips. She complained that everything she ate tasted bad.

There had been enough cases of variant CJD by then that the possibility that Clare had the disease occurred to a neurologist who examined her. The neurologist even discussed the possibility with her family, but they pointed out that Clare was a longtime vegetarian. All the same, in August 1997, doctors took a tonsil biopsy and diagnosed the disease. For some months after that, Clare was in a stable if awful state, howling "like a sick, injured animal," her father remembered. "She looked at you as though you were the devil incarnate. Her eyes were filled with fear. She started to hallucinate." She was incontinent and nearly blind and she had to be tied down toward the end. Mercifully, that came soon, in April 1998.

Clare's death left a new round of questions in an epidemic already full of them. For instance, she had last eaten meat when she was thirteen, in 1985, when supposedly there was no, or at least almost no, BSE in England. Had she just had terrible luck? A more persuasive explanation was that there was far more BSE around far earlier than the government knew. Clare's death was part of a process by which John Wilesmith's epidemiological work was coming under fire. It turned out much of what he had learned was wrong: changes in rendering processes in the mid-1980s would not have left more infectious prions in the bone meal, nor would the removal of powerful solvents have made much of a difference; nor were there more sheep's heads going into feed during the mid-1980s. In other words, if there were infectious prions in cake in 1988, they were probably also there in 1958.

Further studies cast doubt on the assumption that scrapie was the source of the epidemic at all. Molecular studies showed that the BSE prion did not resemble the scrapie prion, at least not after it had been injected into cattle. The BSE prion looked to be a unique, previously unknown strain of prion disease. (It was the USDA that undertook these studies; the British government was less than eager to put to the test the theory that BSE came from sheep.) Had the British government known that BSE might not be "scrapie in a cow," its policies would have been very different. For one thing, it might not have been so content to let its citizens keep eating meat. And if the government had known that BSE had begun, as the new theory suggested, with a cow dying of sporadic CJD on an English farm sometime in the mid-1970s and being sent to a rendering plant, it would have been much better able to prepare for the outbreak—800,000 infected cattle—that hit farms, because it would have known that the infectious agent had already gone through several cycles of infection, slaughter, and reinfection in cattle before it was first noticed a decade later.

There remain many other mysteries still unsolved from the crisis. What started mad cow disease? Why did certain people get sick and others not? Did they eat more meat, or more dangerous kinds? Why are most variant CJD sufferers young? Why has there been more variant CJD in the north of England, while most of the BSE was in the south? Why the 1980s, and why England? (European countries imported massive amounts of contaminated feed from England, yet there were only small mad cow outbreaks on the Continent.) Another lingering mystery is: why are there still BSE cases in Britain, not many, but a few hundred each year? Could the feed bins filled twenty years ago with infectious prions still be contaminated?

For those who participated in those dramatic years, the lack of explanation makes closure difficult. The former MAFF minister John Gummer, for instance, still has not made peace with the events. He keeps asking himself what he did wrong: "Did you look at the evidence that you had? Did you leave anything undone? Did you not do it honestly? Did you not do your work? . . . Did you in any way fail to listen and check on every point?" And Jim Hope, one of the United Kingdom's premier prion researchers, commented: "We were the experts . . . We didn't have many of the answers [but] rather than explain that to a general public, it was thought better to give the impression that we had everything under control, which we didn't and which we never have."

That's not a message very many have heard. In the early years of this century, working on the assumption that mad cow came from scrapie, Europe set about trying to eliminate the "reservoir" for another BSE outbreak by breeding scrapie-resistant sheep. Since then, unfortunately, researchers have discovered that genotypes that confer resistance to most strains of scrapie actually confer susceptibility to others. At the same time, French researchers found that mad cow somehow crossed into a goat. Prions change their shape and their potency as they jump from one species to another, so no one knows whether the resultant goat-BSE prion will also be dangerous to sheep, cattle, humans, or only to goats. Despite our best efforts, we seem more vulnerable than ever.

CHAPTER 12

THE WORLD ACCORDING TO PRIONS

UNITED STATES/BRITAIN, *1970s to present day*

I go to bed every night offering prayers of thanks to the great mad cow in the sky, because it's BSE that has really put our field in the money.

—PAUL BROWN of the NIH

The mad cow epidemic scarred Europe in ways that are still apparent. The European Union ban on most genetically modified foods is evidence of this hurt, as are the speculations that continue on websites as to where prion diseases came from—the insecticide used on cows against warble fly, space dust, a Japanese biological warfare experiment in Papua New Guinea, or an American plot led by Carleton Gajdusek in cahoots with the CIA.*

---

* A 2005 article in *Lancet* suggested that BSE originated in human remains infected with sporadic CJD mixed in with cow protein in India and shipped to the British market for bovine consumption—so, if cows gave humans a prion disease, they were only giving as good as they got.

"This time experts have no answers," the British newspaper *Today* wrote in 1994, after the first probable case of variant CJD was found—and it was true. But by demonstrating how little they understood prion diseases, prion experts paradoxically positioned themselves for an increase in research money to a level they had only dreamed of. With the public furious at their governments for failing to protect them—mad cow was one of the causes of the fall of John Major's government in Britain in 1997—nations invested in prion investigations as they never had before. Worldwide funding went from a pittance to $300 million by the mid-2000s. No one wanted to be caught short a second time.

Some of that money went into getting right the epidemiology of prion diseases; other money went into better understanding the risk posed to humans by infected meat; and much of the rest into improving testing of livestock. But prion researchers also understood that if their work was to matter, it had to have wider applicability. Mad cow, and the sense of urgency it brought, would not be with the world forever. So at the same time as money was going into studies on areas like sheep–cow transmission, many millions of pounds, euros, and dollars were also spent on basic prion science. Prion researchers' hope was to find a place for their discoveries well beyond the infectious and inherited prion diseases that afflict a few thousand people around the globe. They wanted to play a role in curing other diseases and in pioneering innovations in nonbiological fields as well.

That prions might have implications for other diseases was not a new idea. In fact, it was already on Carleton Gajdusek's mind in 1957, when, newly arrived in Papua New Guinea to study kuru, he promised the NIH that if he could "crack" the disease, "parkinsonism, Huntington's chorea, multiple sclerosis, etc., etc." might follow. After he returned to the States and successfully transmitted kuru to chimpanzees in 1965, he tried to make good on his promise, energetically injecting animals with tissue containing other neurological diseases. But of all the neurodegenerative diseases Gajdusek tried to transmit—CJD, multiple sclerosis, ALS, Alzheimer's, Parkinson's, and Huntington's disease, among many others—only CJD proved transmissible. You could not "catch" the others. Gajdusek was enormously disappointed.

When Stanley Prusiner became the leader in prion research, he revived the hope of a world according to prions. Indeed it was a key motive for his renaming the scrapie agent the "prion" in 1982. He was not just trying to get rid of a cumbersome name; he was trying to establish a new disease principle. We say, "He caught a virus" when a person can be suffering from anything from a cold to rabies. Similarly, Prusiner hoped people would say "he has a prion disease," when a person had anything from CJD to—to what?

The list Prusiner drew up included the neurodegenerative disorders that Gajdusek had pursued—Parkinson's disease, Huntington's disease, Alzheimer's disease, MS—and quite a few others, including immune system disorders like Crohn's disease and rheumatoid arthritis and metabolic diseases like adult-onset diabetes.

There has long been anecdotal information suggesting that these diseases have something in common. Many can be inherited but also often just seem to happen by chance. Stress seems to worsen them. The frequency of many increases with age. Jakob thought his patients looked as if they had multiple sclerosis, kuru victims look like Parkinson's sufferers, and the dementia that appears in the prion disease GSS is so similar to Alzheimer's that GSS is almost always first misdiagnosed as the latter. A 1997 paper showed that a Parkinson's drug called Eldepryl (generic name Selegeline) helped patients with moderate Alzheimer's disease, and in 2001 Prusiner's lab published a paper showing that a mutation in the prion gene could cause a prion disease indistinguishable from Huntington's with its characteristic jerky movements, clumsiness, and delusional thinking.

Prusiner and other researchers began to point out in the late 1970s that, besides having overlapping symptoms, all these diseases also left dead, misfolded proteins behind. This shared characteristic was not something researchers who specialized in these ailments had ever paid much attention to. They tended to focus on what was unique to the disease they studied—its symptoms, say, or the absence or excess of a given neurotransmitting chemical. That all these diseases caused the buildup of the same gunk in the body was seen as incidental—an insight no more useful for treatment than, say, the knowledge that many infections leave pus.

By contrast, prion researchers thought the dead, misfolded proteins might be the *cause* of the disease. Most striking to them, most of the diseases produced not just dead, misfolded proteins but dead, misfolded proteins of a particular kind, called amyloid plaques or amyloid fibril sheets. These clumps developed when atoms bonded across the frames of damaged proteins, like the rungs of a fabulously strong ladder. Enzymes couldn't digest them, and water didn't dissolve them. There was nothing in biology as tough; it seemed safe to say that no cell could survive their presence. (Researchers call such structures amyloid because they are white and starchy in appearance, *amylus* being Latin for starch.)

To be sure, the fibrils occurred in different parts of the body in each disease. In Alzheimer's, the clumps of dead protein were in interstitial spaces in the brain; they were so big you could sometimes see them without a microscope. In Parkinson's, the proteins cohered in small, thready masses called Lewy bodies. In Huntington's disease, the dead proteins accumulated in brain neurons. Dead protein clumps didn't have to be in the brain to do damage, either. For instance, in Type II or adult-onset diabetes, the clumps of dead protein built up in the pancreas. In cardiac amyloidosis, they accumulated in the heart, diminishing the organ's ability to pump.

Prion researchers now hoped they could bring the techniques they had honed studying the structures and behaviors of prion proteins to these diseases. The amyloid plaque that most closely resembled a prion was the one found in Alzheimer's disease, so that seemed the logical disease to start with. In the early 1980s, Stanley Prusiner threw his research energies into exploring the overlap between the prion protein and the Alzheimer's protein. (There was more than a little self-interest in the decision: funding for research on the millions of Alzheimer's sufferers was a lot easier to find than funding for prion research.) In prion disease, healthy prion proteins convert to disease-causing ones through a process resembling crystallization: one mis-formed protein touches another, causing it to misform, and so on in a chain reaction. Alzheimer's proteins turn out to be capable of this be-havior, too. If you put a little bit of Alzheimer's amyloid plaque in a test tube with normally formed Alzheimer's proteins, the latter will all eventually refold and bond with the original plaque, forming a single large amyloid plaque. Prusiner thought there was even greater overlap between the two proteins, that, in essence, Alzheimer's were prions, proteins, and he thought he had proven it when, in 1983, working with an Alzheimer's expert, George Glenner of the University of California–San Diego, he showed that both Alzheimer's and prion plaques reacted to the same dye. Dyes are used to tease out the structure of proteins, and the fact that prions and Alzheimer's proteins reacted to the same one suggested that their structures might be identical. Prusiner called the news "astounding"; Glenner, on the other hand, cautioned against leaping to conclusions. "It's like saying two people are related just be-cause they both have red hair," he pointed out.

As researchers learned more about the two diseases over the next few years, distinctions emerged and it became clear that Prusiner's en-thusiasm was excessive. With colleagues he traced the prion to the prion gene on Chromosome 21; Glenner traced his Alzheimer protein to an Alzheimer's protein gene on a different chromosome. The two proteins were composed of different amino acids arranged in a differ-ent sequence. What the researchers had was not a single underlying disease but a single disease principle.

When Prusiner and others returned to amyloid plaques a second time, they did so with broader interests: They wanted to know what they were and how they formed. No two diseases gave the same answer. Researchers went through dozens, from ALS to rheumatoid arthritis to adult-onset diabetes, and identified the key protein that misforms in each of them.

Why proteins form destructive amyloid plaques that injure the cell in the first place is itself an intriguing question. The damage may be a side effect of the general flexibility proteins exhibit: they fold in multiple ways because they have to accomplish many things, and if a physiologically active molecule can fold so many ways, chances are that a few of those ways will be harmful within the small space of a cell. Protein researchers all over the world are working on this problem in their respective diseases today, trying to block proteins from turning into amyloids and amyloids from overwhelming cells. In addition, there are researchers who think that an amyloid does not itself damage the cell but rather protects it by isolating otherwise damaging proteins, restricting them in a bond so strong that, as one protein chemist noted, it is "essentially indestructible under physiological conditions."

Intriguingly, researchers have also verified Gajdusek's old hunch that prions aren't the only transmissible protein—amyloid A amyloidosis, an opportunistic disease that strikes people with chronic inflammations such as rheumatoid arthritis, turns out to share this property. You can inject it into mice and the protein will replicate and the mouse will develop the disease, just as with prions; and the disease can even be transmitted orally. There are also hints that other amyloid plaque diseases such as Alzheimer's can be transmitted—the English prion researchers Rosalind Ridley and Harry Baker reported that they transmitted Alzheimer plaques in 1993. George Glenner, Prusiner's collaborator, died of cardiac amyloidosis in 1995 and, among others, the Alzheimer's researcher Rudolph Tanzi, of Harvard Medical School, wonders whether Glenner may have been infected somehow while working on the protein. If other protein diseases do turn out to be transmissible, it may force researchers to disassemble the boundary between diseases that infect you and diseases that just happen, between those that pursue you and those you acquire by life habits, old age, or environmental toxins. It is possible we will one day talk about people catching MS, Alzheimer's, and even diabetes—or at least a propensity for these diseases.

"The amazing thing is how long it took us to see all these things that were right in front of our face," says Fred Cohen, a molecular chemist at the University of California–San Francisco whose lab works with Prusiner's. "The parallels were obvious."

If prionlike diseases are infectious, though, they are not so in the traditional way. They are not "alive"—infection in their case is purely a mechanical process. The theory of prions threatens to diminish our uniqueness in the universe, which is one reason that—like Galileo's insistence that the earth moves around the sun—it had trouble finding acceptance. It was another example of—in the words of the German chemist Friedrich Wöhler, who discovered in 1828 that he could synthesize the body's chemicals perfectly well in a test tube—"the great tragedy of science, the slaying of a beautiful hypothesis by an ugly fact." The hypothesis was that life is ineffable, uniquely alive; the reality is that it is just chemical. Or, as Justus von Liebig wrote in 1855, life is nothing more than "chemical processes dependent upon common chemical forces."

It should not be surprising then that a branch of biology that traces disease to nonliving, mechanical processes had also turned out to be useful in engineering. Chemists are familiar with conformational influence, which they call nucleation. Briefly, nucleation is the tendency of molecules to arrange themselves, typically in an orderly fashion, around a first fixed point: this process gives material remarkable strength. Silk

is a product of nucleation, and so is the abalone shell, its nacreous surface three thousand times stronger than if it were made of nonnucleated
material. In fact, J. S. Griffith got the idea that would turn out to be the
basis of prion theory from mechanical physics, from the way checkers,
if shaken on a checkerboard with one checker in a fixed position, will
assume an orderly pattern around the original checker. The prion researcher Byron Caughey co-authored an interesting paper on nucleation in 1995, in which he compared prions to Ice-9. Ice-9, an invention
of the novelist Kurt Vonnegut in his novel *Cat's Cradle,* is a variant of
water that freezes at a higher temperature. In the novel, a madman deliberately releases Ice-9 seeds, which, through nucleation, cause all the
water in the world to freeze. (Vonnegut got his ideas from his brother
Bernard, who is credited with discovering cloud seeding to increase
rainfall, another example of nucleation.)

Papers like Caughey's and novels like Vonnegut's suggest how se-
ductive nucleation is to the imagination, one reason it has attracted
Carleton Gajdusek. Gajdusek's mind continued to be fertile, even during his time in jail. He enjoyed incarceration, in fact; he loved how simple it made his life, never having to know where his wallet was or which
of his clothes were clean. "No hotel could offer more punctual and po-
lite service," he wrote in his journal in 1997. The warden let him do his
work in the common room after lights out, and his personal writings
blossomed. "At the rate I am going, 1997 will be the most verbose journal of my life," he noted happily in its pages.

The government released Gajdusek on five years' probation in
1998, with permission to serve the time abroad. Then seventy-four, he
had gained an enormous amount of weight; his brother described him
as looking like "a great Buddha." Once unstoppable, as he trekked
through the Highland jungles, he now had trouble walking. He went
directly to his lawyer's office, got his passport, had a party at Dulles
Airport with friends (among them several other Nobelists), and flew to

France. "He wishes to roll around among different labs like Diogenes in a barrel," one European scientist said at the time.

Gajdusek, who now lives in Amsterdam, is content in his exile. He is open—obsessive—about his long-hidden sexuality. "I am a pedagogic pedophiliac pediatrician," he greeted me in 2003 when I called to arrange a meeting. Mostly he spends his time reading and thinking about big ideas, the sort that always appealed to him more than lab work.

One subject of his inquiry is how life-forms can replicate without DNA. According to Gajdusek: "life is nucleation, conformational change, and replication." At the same time, so is nonlife. He asks whether nucleating forces explain the arrangement of stars in a galaxy, and whether fossils could serve as templates for the re-creation of vanished life-forms.

Among the other questions that interest Gajdusek is the mystery of why prions—or "nucleating amyloids," as he calls them, still resisting Prusiner's term—are so hard to disinfect. The probability that prions have no DNA cannot really explain this robustness: even prion *ash* is infectious. Gajdusek theorizes that there is a nanoscopic bit of clay or silica in the prion that captures the form of the protein after the rest of the structure has been incinerated. These molecular templates— "atomic ghost replicas," in Gajdusek's words—wait for new intact prions that will adapt to their shape to begin the infection cycle again. "In this case," Gajdusek wrote in a 2001 paper, "we can really speak of the fantasy of a 'virus' from the inorganic world."

Self-assembling biological systems like protein plaques and nonbiological ones like crystals are a new frontier, and many researchers have taken up the challenge. One is a professor of biomedical engineering at MIT named Shuguang Zhang. Zhang is an unabashed disciple of Gajdusek; he keeps a blow-up of the Nobel laureate on his shelf. Zhang is trying to put nucleation to work in medicine. Biology has always lacked a modeling mechanism that is more complicated than a petri dish, in which experiments are easy to execute but not very true to life, but less complicated than a living animal, in which experiments are true to life but hard to execute. Zhang is using nucleation to create a third way. He has developed watery protein solutions that can form three-dimensional scaffolds. He has also shown how these scaffolds can speed healing when injected into the body, functioning like dissolving stitches, and other times how they can enter the body, organize to open a cell wall, and then dissolve to allow it to close again after a medication bonded to the molecules has entered. These two examples are only the beginning of what self-assembling proteins might accomplish in medicine, according to Zhang. Colleagues are trying to zap molecules with radio transmitters to get them to assume different shapes in the body. They hope one day to persuade stem cells on scaffoldings to grow into muscles or neurons.

There are plenty of potential applications for self-assembling systems outside the body as well—tiny systems using the forces of nucleation could be useful for everything from plastics that build themselves to tiny circuits that can assemble themselves at the molecular level, on a computer chip. The trick, according to Zhang, is to appropriate the work nature has already done—to glean the secrets of the tiny machine that is the cell and co-opt its genius to one's own purposes. Opposition has already sprung up to self-assembling systems too, the worry being that we have no idea how safe any of this technology is and what its effect on our bodies or the environment may be. Opponents point to the Buckyball, a self-assembling, soccer ball–shaped carbon nanomolecule. Once thought to be harmless, it now turns out to persist in the environment for considerable time when released, invading the cells of living things with unknown consequences. We tap the power of the cell at our peril, though Zhang is not worried. "We have had the Stone Age, the Bronze Age, and the plastic age," he says. "The future is the designed material age."

CHAPTER 13

DID MAN EAT MAN? WORLDWIDE, *800,000 B.C.E.*

The pursuit of the prion disease mystery has been in many ways a study in frustrations, in long experiments that went nowhere and high hopes that were not borne out. Nature is sometimes too original to be understood through paradigms, and presents puzzles too complicated to be solved on a human time scale. But for all their frustrations, prion researchers also solved an old anthropological puzzle.

Anthropologists have long debated whether humans are cannibalistic. The question is not whether humans ever eat human flesh—clearly we sometimes do when the alternative is starvation—but whether cannibalism was ever central to a human culture. Over the centuries, that assertion was made many times and in regards to many cultures. The Fore, the Anga, and the Mundugumor of New Guinea; the Fijians of the South Seas; the Aztecs, the Arawaks, and the Caribs of the New World ("cannibal" derives from the word "Carib") are but a few of the peoples whom neighbors, travelers, and, later, Western anthropologists claimed regularly ate human flesh, either to honor their dead, to avenge their enemies, or simply for the nutrition. Yet it turned out that on closer examination there were never firsthand accounts to confirm these stories. Most travelers' accounts were derived from previous travelers' accounts, themselves secondhand and probably distorted. Anthropologists, in turn, got a lot of their information from local hearsay. As one skeptical anthropologist wrote in 1979, "The human failing which emerges most clearly from the morass of data is . . . European plagiarism."

Even the kuru epidemic can be explained without cannibalism. Gajdusek has long maintained that the handling of infected bodies in preparation for burial would have been sufficient to spread the disease. And though the early Highland patrol reports are full of comments that the Fore considered themselves cannibals, eyewitness accounts are not to be found. "If opportunity presents itself I propose to avail myself of an invitation extended by a Kagu leader to be present at some future ceremonial eating of human flesh to observe the various rites practiced," promises the first patrol officer to enter Fore territory, R. I. Skinner, in the late 1940s. But the opportunity never does present itself.

So a generation of anticannibalism anthropologists have been able to gain traction, arguing that to call a tribe "cannibalistic" is not descriptive, but pejorative.

That is no longer true. Without deliberately setting out to settle the point, an effort in England to understand why some Britons got sick from mad cow disease while others didn't has proven that cannibalism was part of early human history. In fact, not only were we all cannibals at one point, but it cost us dearly: our anthropophagy led to an outbreak of a prion disease with a high death toll (and probably caused us to evolve a tendency to feel revulsion at the act that made cannibalism, in more recent history, taboo.)

This important discovery by prion investigators began in the 1980s soon after the prion gene was found. They were interested in why some mammals seemed particularly susceptible to prion disease—say, certain breeds of sheep—while others were resistant. They wondered whether there was something in the sheep's genetic makeup that affected its chances of coming down with scrapie if it was exposed to the infectious agent.

Over time it became clear that susceptibility to prion diseases often depends on small alterations in an animal's prion gene. Genes contain the blueprints, or recipes, for all the proteins in the body. Most mammals have the same genes for the same proteins as other members of their species, but fairly often there are two or more genetic codes that result in essentially the same protein. These variations are called polymorphisms. The human genome is full of them, and they often have little or no effect on their possessors.

In the early 1990s, the English prion researcher John Collinge undertook a prion gene analysis of Britons to see if a similar relationship existed between a polymorphism and susceptibility to prion disease in the human population. This was before there were any human mad cow victims, but there existed a group of young CJD sufferers whom I have not mentioned yet: teenagers who had gotten CJD from growth hormone derived from human pituitary glands. From the 1950s to the 1980s, British doctors gave the hormones to eighteen hundred children, a few of whom developed CJD, because the donor cadavers had it and the preparation of the injection did not remove the infectious prions. The first such case was reported in the mid-1980s; by the time mad cow was first suspected among beef eaters, there were six human growth hormone CJD sufferers in the United Kingdom.

Collinge found an interesting pattern in the group infected by pituitary growth hormone: four had the same polymorphism on their prion genes. He then looked at sufferers of sporadic CJD, and found an even higher ratio: out of forty-five sporadic CJD sufferers, forty had the combination. These forty, like the four human growth hormone recipients, each had the genetic code for an amino acid called valine in a key spot on each of their two prion genes (every human has two copies of every gene, one from each parent). They were what is called homozygous for valine.

Collinge needed to know the overall British genetic makeup to see whether the percentage of homozygous growth hormone CJD victims and sporadic CJD victims was unusual. It was, after all, possible that there were just a lot of British people walking around with that particular genotype. But surveying British genetic data, Collinge found the reverse—Britons with a valine on each copy of their prion gene were scarcer in the population than chance would dictate. Collinge's lab thus concluded that homozygosity somehow left the carrier more susceptible to prion disease.

It was important for Collinge to make sure that this pattern also held for susceptibility to infection under natural conditions, because CJD born of an injection often behaves differently from CJD that originates outside the laboratory. There was a place to see a human natural infectious prion disease in action: Papua New Guinea. Skeptics could argue over whether Papua New Guinea had been the site of cannibalism, but no one could argue about its being the site of a prion disease epidemic. In the years after mad cow disease was discovered, the territory had become a de facto laboratory for seeing how this rare epidemiological event played out. Elderly Papua New Guinean women were still dying from prion infections contracted at burial feasts they had participated in forty years before.

Collinge's prion unit was in touch with Michael Alpers, Gajdusek's old researcher, who still ran the kuru research program in Okapa. The British researchers asked Alpers to take blood samples from some survivors of the feasts. Of the thirty women Alpers tested, only seven were homozygotes; the twenty-three others had one valine and one of another amino acid that can substitute for valine called methionine at the site of their polymorphism. They were heterozygous. Their heterozygosity likely had helped them survive: the number was too high to be coincidental. In fact, the blood tests of living Fore showed that they had the highest percentage of heterozygotes of anyone in the world. The inescapable conclusion was that they had had some sort of protection from kuru.

Because of Collinge's work, many prion researchers suspected that if mad cow crossed over to humans it too would attack homozygotes disproportionately. And when it did, in the mid-1990s, they were proven right. By 2003 the plague was almost a decade old and the number of people dead from variant CJD (the human form of mad cow) was around 150. If, as has been estimated, the English were exposed to 640 billion doses of mad cow, they had done a remarkable job of surviving the onslaught. This was a tragedy, certainly, but why weren't more people dying?

The main answer was that the prion crossed species only with difficulty. Human prions infect humans quite well—viz. kuru—and cows do the same for cows—viz. mad cow disease. That's because prion contamination is a physical event. It is necessary for the two proteins to fit together well for the disease to spread. The more different the proteins of the infector and the host, the less likely transmission is; the more similar, the more likely. That's why the most alarming prion outbreaks have begun with same-species infection.

But that didn't answer the question of why BSE seemed to cross to some humans more easily than others. Collinge found that the striking pattern he saw at the beginning of the epidemic was even more remarkable now: all but one of the victims of mad cow in Britain to date was a homozygote (they all had two methionines on their prion gene). This pattern suggested, happily, that a good many of the Britons had some degree of resistance to mad cow disease, because the majority of them were heterozygotes.

In 2004, Collinge's group received laboratory data to back up their theory: they created mice with homozygous human prion genes, challenged them with mad cow prions, and found they were more likely to become infected with BSE than mice with heterozygous human prion genes. There was something in heterozygosity that altered the shape of the prion to make it less effective at spreading within the body. (Elio Lugaresi and Pierluigi Gambetti in the late 1990s found a parallel pattern with the fast and slow forms of FFI; Assunta and Silvano were homozygotes and died quickly. Luigia and Teresa were heterozygotes; their disease course was much longer.) In addition, heterozygosity may play a role in the recently discovered phenomenon of healthy prion mutation carriers: For years, researchers believed that everyone who had a prion gene mutation ultimately got the disease, but more recent research shows that there are people who have a prion mutation but never get sick, or at least die of old age–related diseases before they get sick. Possibly heterozygosity is giving them some degree of protection.

Collinge and his lab had now identified an important epidemiological pattern: homozygotes were at higher risk of prion disease than heterozygotes and there were more heterozygotes in the British population than chance would dictate. The researchers speculated that the two facts might be connected—some evolutionary force might have favored heterozygotes over homozygotes.

That made what the lab learned next particularly intriguing: heterozygotes were overrepresented worldwide, in every race and every ethnicity. According to the theory of population genetics, then, their common ancestors must have faced a situation that winnowed out the homozygotes. To have altered so many genomes, it would have had to be a severe challenge to human survivability and it would either have had to happen all across the earth or to have arisen very early in human history when humans lived only in Africa.

Collinge and his lab set out to put an estimated date on this mysterious event. With the help of a population geneticist, they were able to establish the history of this portion of the prion gene; they found that methionine was the original amino acid coded for on the prion gene and that valines started to appear in the same position around 500,000 years ago. New amino acids can appear and hang around for hundreds of millennia without purpose, so long as they do no harm, so Collinge's dating can be taken only as the earliest possible occurrence of whatever event had thinned out the homozygotes in favor of the heterozygotes.

Most paleoanthropologists believe modern humanity comes from a small group of *Homo sapiens* who lived in Africa around seventy thousand years ago. These humans may have numbered no more than two thousand. If so, a quite small number of humans would have needed to engage in some behavior that changed the balance of methionine and valine in their prion protein. But what was the behavior? To figure it out, Collinge and his team had to think about the lives our distant ancestors lived.

Humans of this era were quite healthy (average life span actually declined when humans first began to form agricultural settlements around ten thousand years ago). They died mostly from accidents and, during periods of famine, from malnutrition. They had little experience with infectious diseases, and as a result, very little resistance to them. So if you wanted to kill a lot of early humans, you couldn't choose a better way than a novel infectious disease.

But what kind of disease? The most successful contagions among humans at this time were slow-acting ones. That's because when land is thickly populated, virulent infections prosper. There are sufficient hosts: burn one out, move on to the next (the measles virus, for instance, needs 300,000 people and 3,000 infections a year to keep going; it needs cities to prosper). But in preagricultural times, with humans so spread out, an infection had to have a very mild degree of aggressiveness to hitch a ride from one host to the next. Otherwise it killed its victims faster than it could find new ones.

What would be the optimal vector for this infection? Perhaps meat. Food, in general, is an ideal way to get a pathogen into people's bodies, because they seek it out and put it in their own mouths. And we know people ate meat in prehistory; they had grown too large to subsist entirely on fruit, berries, and wild grains, and needed concentrated protein. And meat is an excellent source of pathogens. Given that ancient peoples had no drugs to treat infection, it would not be surprising to find a huge mortality rate from a food-borne illness at the time.

Arguing against meat as the source of this ancient plague are two factors. One, stomach acids do a good job of removing infectivity; and, two, early on humans learned to cook what they ate. Meat is far less dangerous when it is cooked, because heating kills bacteria. The first confirmed evidence for fire only dates back to around 150,000 B.C.E., but there are several hints that hominids mastered it before they switched from the vegetarianism of their ancestors. For one thing, the climate of northern Europe required fire for survival, given the extreme cold of periodic glaciations. Embers don't fossilize well, so the absence of hearths in earlier sites is not necessarily unexpected. The argument is a bit circular—we know there was fire because hominids had grown so large they needed meat—but it has some validity.

So, in this prehuman population posited by Collinge and his colleagues—spread around the world, able to use fire and to hunt, beset by no known conventional disease—a successful contagion would be one that infected its victims very slowly. If it was in meat it would have to survive aggressive stomach acids and extensive cooking. And it would have to come from a source of meat that was readily available to humans everywhere. The meat that best meets these criteria would have been human flesh, and the act that would best spread any disease-causing agent in flesh would be cannibalism.

How much cannibalism would have had to occur to spread a prehistoric prion plague across the world? If the experience of the Fore is an indication, not much. Kuru likely started with a single sporadic CJD case, probably early in the twentieth century. That person's relatives and friends ate him or her at a mortuary feast and, after they fell ill and died, they were in turn eaten by their relatives and friends. Within fifty years, an epidemic severe enough to kill half the residents of some villages was underway.

But what about the initial doubt I mentioned, that cannibalism caused kuru at all? What about the theory held by Gajdusek that handling the tissues of the dead was enough for a prion disease to spread? This objection wouldn't apply to an ancient prion plague. The first human burial ceremonies date from around fifty thousand years ago, hundreds of thousands of years after the protective polymorphism likely began spreading. There is no evidence that early hominids buried their dead, but there is a lot of evidence that they ate them.

Atapuerca is an important archaeological site in northern Spain. A series of hillside caves overlooking a river valley, it has attracted animals and humans looking for shelter since ancient times. Many of these animals and humans died there too, so Atapuerca presents a kind of smorgasbord of remains. Its five or six dig sites each correspond to a different epoch of prehistory. One is Gran Dolina, a site uncovered at the end of the nineteenth century that contains prehuman remains. Archaeologists have been able to date the site back to roughly 800,000 B.C.E., when the earth's magnetic field last switched. This makes Gran Dolina the oldest repository of hominid remains in Europe.

Two of the hominid remains discovered at Gran Dolina were the bodies of a fourteen-year-old and a ten-year-old, found at the mouth of the cave. That's a noteworthy location, because the mouth of a cave is where animals normally eat their prey. It occurred to the archaeologists involved that some prehistoric animal seized these children and consumed them in the cave's shady entrance—carnivores, among them bear and hyena, were abundant in the area. But further research showed that the children's bones, as well as some animal bones found nearby, were dissected with a precision that exceeds the skills of non-human carnivores: for instance, two segments of finger or toe bone and a cranium had the meat scraped out of them. Other bones had been snapped so the marrow could be sucked out. Stone flints were found lying near the remains. Two scenarios might explain what went on at Gran Dolina. Either hominids celebrated some sort of ritual that involved pulling the meat off their dead, or, more probably (because hominids of 800,000 years ago were unlikely to be capable of such symbolic behavior) they were eating other hominids for food.

The official Atapuerca website speculates that "for these primitive humans the difference between the body of a deer and a human cadaver didn't exist yet." That's an evasive statement—even chimpanzees recognize their own kind, so let's assume at least a similar level of cultural sophistication among the Atapuerca hominids. The bones of the ten-year-old show evidence of malnutrition. Maybe there was a series of bad hunts in the area, or a drought, and the lack of vegetation drove the large herbivores away. It is easy to imagine how urgently the hominids needed some meat. Maybe they attacked and killed their own children, but again, chimpanzees don't do that, so we can assume hominids didn't. It's more likely that the children died of starvation and the parents thought: Why waste this? Especially with other mouths to feed? In the words of the Fore man recorded by anthropologists more than three quarters of a million years later: "What is the matter with us, are we mad? Here is good food and we have neglected to eat it."

So, using a blade made by sharpening one stone against another, the parents sliced off one of their children's legs. They cracked the long part of the femur and gave the nutritious marrow to their surviving offspring. They worked their way through the large muscles of the body, then struck open the skull and removed what was inside and ate that. Done, they threw the human bones at their feet among the deer bones and the pony bones left from more flush times. They were not capable of reflecting on whether what they had done was wrong or right, but emotional pain precedes morality; they may have cried; they may have agonized, but at the same time would have known that what they were doing was the obligatory thing in order for their family to survive.

This is all possible. But of course it also may be wrong. Maybe one clan ambushed another. Maybe they ate the enemy's dead to intimidate the survivors. A ritual ingestion of one's defeated rivals is well known in anthropology. Chimpanzees even do it. And the hominids at Gran Dolina are our ancestors, as well as those of the Neanderthals. We know that of those two groups one, our own, with which these hominids shared nearly all their genes, shows little compunction against war and murder. We don't know whether intentional killing led to the feast in the mouth of the cave at Gran Dolina. Probably we never will. The one thing that never survives in the fossil record is motive. But whatever the cause, amazingly, 800,000 years later, this behavior that cost them so dearly and began to turn the human race against cannibalism forever saved our lives.

Skeptical anthropologists will have to update their ideas as Collinge and his colleagues' proof sinks in. But they will have some consolation. Their main objection to the charge of cannibalism was that Europeans used it to justify their racism. For instance, the Spanish in destroying Aztec civilization made clear that the savages they wiped out were eaters of human flesh and thus not worthy of compassion. They were not alone in this assumption. The Aztecs, too, believed in cannibals. In fact, the figure of the cannibal played a central role in their mythic life. They thought the Indians to the north and the south were cannibals (with cannibalism it is always the other guy who does it). And when Cortés and his soldiers arrived, they thought a new cannibal tribe had come to attack them. That was why they fought so hard when they saw the Spanish. It turns out they were right after all: at Gran Dolina are the remains of the first Europeans, and already they were eating each other.

CHAPTER 14

COMING TO AMERICA?

UNITED STATES, *present day*

U.S. beef is safe, plain and simple. . . . I enjoyed beef
this noon for lunch.

> —MIKE JOHANNS, U.S. secretary of agriculture,
> after the announcement of the second case of mad
> cow discovered in America in June 2005

One day Carrie Mahan, a twenty-nine-year-old woman from a town outside of Philadelphia, was fine. The next she could barely walk and couldn't unlock her car door. At a hospital emergency room in Philadelphia in January 2000 doctors gave her medicine and suggested rest. But she was back the next day, complaining of anxiety, nausea, and hallucinations. This time, she was admitted. Things got worse quickly. She faded in and out of consciousness and her legs began to jerk. Then she fell into a coma and was put on life support.

About a month later, on February 24, 2000, doctors took the tubes out of her mouth and nose and veins and she was allowed to die.

Early on, one of Mahan's neurologists, Peter Crino, had written in her chart, "Could this be CJD?" The possibility struck him as unlikely because Creutzfeldt-Jakob disease is rare, and even rarer in twenty-nine-year-olds. So the working diagnosis was a viral infection of the brain. When Crino saw Carrie's lab results, though, he thought again about CJD. The inquest on Victoria Rimmer, the English girl whose sickness in 1993 was the first probable case of mad cow in a human, described her brain as like that of "a 90-year-old woman who had undergone severe neurological damage." Crino saw something similar in Mahan's brain tissue. "She had holes all over the place," he remembered. "She clearly had a devastating neurologic injury. Her brain was just gone."

Crino and the pathologist he worked with, Nicholas Gonatas, were not sure what to make of the death. A genetic form of Creutzfeldt-Jakob disease or Gerstmann-Sträussler-Scheinker disease, rather than a sporadic one, was most likely, given Carrie's youth. But she did not have a history of the disease in her family. She had received no growth hormone injections and had never been to England, making the possibility of infection from food remote. So Crino and Gonatas settled for a diagnosis of sporadic CJD.

Allen Mahan, her brother, was skeptical. He was sure, even before she died, that she had variant CJD. He had read up on the human form of mad cow disease. The mad cow victims in Britain had been young. They had had symptoms of psychiatric disturbance. His sister had been mentally unstable when she first arrived at the hospital, disoriented and making advances at the doctors. Allen Mahan got Crino to call Robert Will at the CJD surveillance unit in Edinburgh, where the key work on mad cow and variant CJD had been done, to ask for a second opinion on what had killed Carrie. Will said the rapidity of Carrie's death and her genetic makeup—she did not have the methionine-

methionine polymorphism found in all variant CJD victims to date—made variant CJD unlikely. Allen Mahan had no choice but to accept the hospital's diagnosis of sporadic CJD, even if the likelihood of getting sporadic CJD is one in a million. That Carrie was African-American made CJD even less likely—more like 1 in 2.5 million, and that she was only twenty-nine made the odds longer still.

There turned out to be yet another problem with the sporadic-CJD diagnosis. Crino and Gonatas had sent some of Mahan's brain tissue to Pierluigi Gambetti, the nation's leading prion disease pathologist, at Case Western Reserve. When Gambetti subjected Carrie's tissue to prion antibody tests, to everyone's surprise the antibody did not react, meaning it did not recognize the protein as a prion. Gonatas, an old teacher of Gambetti's, wasn't convinced. He urged Gambetti, "Try it again." He did, and the test came back negative again.

The diagnosis of prion diseases has come a long way since the days when British researchers had to shoot scrapie into mice and wait years to see if the animal got sick, but it is still an unstable body of knowledge. Sometimes the prions are only located in discrete parts of the brain and the test misses them; other times there aren't enough of them to trigger a positive result. Still, Gambetti has confidence that the combination of tests he subjects tissue to will find even hard-to-spot cases. He believed Carrie had died of some other disease whose symptoms resembled CJD and was not surprised at the lack of an antibody response since 40 percent of the cases referred to him as CJD test negative for prions.

But Carrie's family and friends did not accept this nonanswer. They continued to agitate for the diagnosis to be revisited, and four years after her death, Gambetti pulled out slides of Carrie's brain tissue and tested it again. By then, the urgency of knowing whether Carrie died of mad cow disease had intensified, because the federal government had acknowledged America's first mad cow.

—

Most Americans didn't much care about mad cow disease when it struck Britain in the 1980s. While Europeans tended to blame their epidemic on American-style agribusiness, Americans watching the images of burning English cows on the nightly news regarded them as ghoulish dispatches from the Old World. America had led the world in production safety since the days of Theodore Roosevelt; the U.S. Department of Agriculture inspection stamp was as familiar—and as reassuring— as the *Good Housekeeping* Seal of Approval.

The USDA was similarly unworried about mad cow. After the epidemiologist John Wilesmith traced the disease to infected meat and bone meal in Britain in 1988, the agency found to its satisfaction that the United States was not a significant importer of British feed. American ranchers had imported several hundred British cattle for breeding in recent years; the USDA located half of them (it could not find the rest) and eventually bought them for slaughter. Because most were beef cattle, not dairy cattle, and thus less likely to have mad cow, the agency soon after declared America mad cow free. For the $27 billion beef industry, that was very good news.

But a few Americans were not reassured. They weren't convinced the USDA had done what it could to protect them. They knew that the agency's image as a protector of consumers was part myth, because the USDA, just like the Ministry of Agriculture, Fisheries and Food, its counterpart in Britain, had another important—and contradictory— role. Besides looking after the safety of food, it also looked after the health of the food industries. In the past twenty years that role had become paramount.

The Reagan Revolution, with its emphasis on letting businesses do business, essentially pulled the plug on government inspectors and their authority. Today meat companies run their own inspection systems, while USDA inspectors mostly examine the records of the companies for compliance. Affidavits from USDA meat inspectors give the impression that slaughterhouses have become places where the inspector is not only outmanned by company personnel but also receives demoralizing responses from his own superiors if he tries to do his or her job. Meat covered with feces, deformed by abscesses, or dropped on the floor and hung back up on the assembly line is common, according to these inspectors' testimony. One result is an increasing occurrence of food-borne sickness: 5,000 deaths a year and 200,000 cases of food poisoning a *day,* according to the Centers for Disease Control.

The people I call the Creutzfeldt Jakobins—those worried about mad cow disease in America, food activists, vegetarians, organic meat buyers, nearly anyone who has had a relative die of a neurodegenerative disease whose diagnosis did not satisfy their family—did not forget that when mad cow was first discovered in Britain, the government there all but covered it up to protect the beef and milk markets. The Creutzfeldt Jakobins expected the same behavior from the USDA, should a mad cow turn up.

In the mid-1990s, more to reassure foreign markets than to calm any anxious Americans, the USDA announced that it would begin testing cattle for mad cow disease. It would focus the program on cows that could not walk when they got to the slaughterhouse—known as downer or "four D" (dead, dying, disabled, or diseased) cattle; downers were thought to present the highest risk of prion disease. (In Britain, even before BSE, downer cattle were never allowed to enter the human food chain.)

The USDA didn't say how many cows it would test. Roughly 35 million cattle are slaughtered each year in the United States, and, it turned out, the USDA planned to test only about one in a thousand (by comparison, European countries consistently test almost 25 percent of their cows). In defending this number, the USDA explained that its goal was not to catch a mad cow before Americans ate it but to take a sampling of the American cattle population to see whether mad cow was a significant problem. All forty thousand tests came back negative.

Then in late December 2003, the USDA announced that a downer cow from a Washington herd had tested positive. It emphasized its surprise, though it had long been bruited among prion researchers that there would be some cases of mad cow in the U.S. cattle population— if only because until 1997 the United States had allowed cow and sheep protein in American cow feed (including until 1989 *British* meat and bone meal). Much to the agency's relief, a few days later, the cow turned out to be more than six years old, meaning it was born before the 1997 ban on feeding sheep and cow protein to cows was put in place. To the USDA's even greater relief, the cow also turned out to have been born in Canada. "This puts a different perspective on things," the USDA's chief veterinary officer said at a news conference, barely containing his delight. The problem wasn't an American one at all.

Yet the world didn't buy this line: Japan, America's biggest importer of beef, embargoed it (Japan is terrified of BSE because its population's genetic makeup is heavily homozygous) and more than forty countries followed Japan's example.

To try to restore overseas confidence in American beef, Ann Veneman, then the secretary of agriculture, announced that her agency would begin testing ten times as many cattle as before. She simultaneously rallied domestic eaters to the table: "We see no need for people to alter . . . their eating habits or to do anything but have a happy and healthy holiday season," she said at a news conference on December 23. "I plan to serve beef for my Christmas dinner, and we remain confident in the safety of our food supply." So then why increase the number of tests at all? "An abundance of caution," Veneman said, as if channeling the MAFF ministers in Britain who had walked this road almost a decade before.

There was, though, such a thing as being too cautious. When a small Kansas beef producer announced its intention to satisfy the Japanese by testing *all* its cattle, the USDA blocked the move. The agency's motive was obvious: confidence in American beef depended on *not* knowing what risk it presented. Enormous amounts of money were at stake—for instance, Tyson Foods, the huge meat producer, potentially stood to double its profits if the international ban on American beef were removed. The case of the Kansas beef producer drew coverage throughout the world and was widely followed by the e-mail lists of consumer food safety groups in America, who once again drew parallels between the early days of mad cow in England and the events occurring now in America.

Nothing about the USDA's behavior inspired confidence. Every time it proposed to toughen mad cow controls, beef industry groups—who held many key posts in the agency—quietly reached out and reversed the proposal. Fifty billion tons of livestock were processed in the country every year and no one seemed to have the political power to make it safer. Veneman herself was a former lobbyist who had served on the board of a company called Calgene, makers of the Flavr Savr tomato, the first genetically modified food for sale to consumers. That she had been present at the creation of "Frankenfood" was not lost on the Creutzfeldt Jakobins.

A later near miss on the mad cow front increased consumer doubt. In April 2004 a deranged cow in Texas was destroyed after a regional inspector overruled a department veterinarian who wanted to test it, and then in January 2005, the Canadians discovered a cow with BSE that had been born *after* the animal-protein feed bans that both that country and the United States had put in place in 1997. It was now likely that, just as it had been in Britain, the feed ban was leaking. There were plenty of anecdotes to that effect: stories of mills that weren't properly separating cow protein from pig protein; ranchers who, to save money, kept feeding cow and sheep protein to their cows after the ban.

One fact about the December 2003 Washington mad cow particularly unsettled Creutzfeldt Jakobins. The USDA said the cow in question was a downer. But three of the four individuals who saw the cow at the slaughterhouse said it was walking and had only been classified as a downer because a slaughterhouse worker, seeing the cow flailing as it approached, killed it so it wouldn't trample other cattle in the trailer. The dispute prompted the USDA's inspector general to begin an investigation. Her conclusion would be important: if the cow was *walking* and had BSE, and the USDA had been testing only downers, it had not been testing enough cows.

Creutzfeldt Jakobins seized on two widely cited research studies that might shed light on this important question. In the first study, performed in the early 1990s, Richard Marsh, a researcher at the University of Wisconsin who trained with Carleton Gajdusek, and the scrapie researcher William Hadlow, took prion disease–infected mink, injected their tissue into healthy cattle, and found that, though the cattle got a prion disease, the disease did not look like BSE in Britain. The pattern of holes and plaques in the cows' brains was different. Another difference was that when the cows were about to die, they just collapsed. Before that, they showed no signs of sickness.

The other paper was by the husband and wife team of Elias and Laura Manuelidis, professors of neurology at Yale. In the late 1980s, the Manuelidises' lab sampled tissue from forty-six patients whose death certificates said they'd died of Alzheimer's but were otherwise chosen at random. The lab found that six of the forty-six had actually died of CJD. Later studies paralleled the Manuelidises' findings. Because several million Americans have Alzheimer's, these studies opened up the possibility that several thousand people could be dying of CJD every year without the medical community's noticing.

The two papers came to the fore again when the USDA announced that there was a second mad cow in June 2005. This cow, a downer, tested positive in a rapid screening test, but when the USDA followed up with what it called its "gold-standard" test, that came back negative. Then the USDA tested the animal a third time with a positive result but took no action because it considered the testing technique experimental. Then, the USDA's inspector general went around the secretary of agriculture and ordered the much-sampled cow tested a fourth time. Again the test came out positive. Finally, the USDA sent samples to a British testing lab, where the animal was confirmed to have BSE, roughly seven months after it was slaughtered. An announcement had to be made. Unlike the Washington State cow found almost a year and a half before, this cow had been born in America, which was bad, but it was old enough to have been born before the ruminant feed ban, which was good. The bigger worry was that its prion infection seemed irregular, much as the ones Richard Marsh had noted in the mid-1980s were irregular. That the animal had tested negative with the USDA's best test also raised the possibility that the agency was using a test that did not detect the strain of prion disease that American cows actually had.

All the same, the USDA congratulated itself: the animal had not gotten into the food supply, and finding just one more positive result among the now more than 400,000 tests was heartening. Mike Johanns, the replacement for Ann Veneman (who had gone off to be executive director of UNICEF), declared U.S. beef to be "safe, plain and simple. . . . I enjoyed beef this noon for lunch. It is the safest in the world, and I will continue to enjoy beef." He assured the press he was telling it "like it is."

Johanns did not try to explain what had prompted the USDA's inspector general to request a retest of a retest of two initial tests, or—as later came out—why the cow's failing an earlier test had not been part of an earlier report filed on the cow ("The laboratory folks just never mentioned it to anyone higher up," a USDA spokesman explained).

Taiwan, having just reopened its doors to American beef two months before, shut them again, and Tyson Foods' shares lost 3 percent the next business day.

After the second cow, the USDA ramped up testing still further, going on to test more than half a million sick or dead cows. Japan, heavily pressured by America, reopened its borders to American beef in December 2005, only to close them again a few weeks later when it found to its horror that a U.S. meat packer had accidentally shipped them spinal tissue. A report that downer cattle were still getting into beef shipments—downers were supposed to have been banned after the Washington State cow of December 2003—got wide circulation there, too, and "might further fuel anger of Japanese government and consumers," as the newspaper *Yomiuri Shimbun* warned. And even as the USDA continued to assure the public that American beef was safe and announced it would begin to curtail its testing program, a third U.S. mad cow was found in March 2006 in Alabama and another Canadian cow born after the feed ban was found in April. At times it felt like all that was missing was the Oinkies.

When they consider whether mad cow has crossed over to the U.S. human population, Creutzfeldt Jakobins turn their attention to CJD. Basically, they do not believe CJD ever just happens by chance. They believe instead that what scientists call sporadic CJD is really variant CJD (mad cow disease in humans) and that the government just refuses to acknowledge the fact, out of incompetence or duplicity. In other words, as they see it, mad cow is already in America and killing people; we just don't know it.

Throughout the first half of the decade, a Texan named Terry Singeltary was the most visible member of this group. Wiry, with his hair in a silvery ponytail, Singeltary is a self-described "redneck hippie" and a high-school dropout. He lost his mother to a fast form of

Creutzfeldt-Jakob disease called the Heidenhain variant in 1997. The variant blinds the patient by hollowing out a part of the brain that connects to the optic nerve. After this horror, Singeltary found out that, exactly a year earlier, the mother of his next-door neighbor in tiny Bacliff, Texas, had died of CJD too. After that, he began educating himself on the disease, taking particular note of the Marsh paper on the possibility of a domestic strain of BSE. It all made him look at the USDA's food safety policies with new eyes. Today he believes that his mother was infected by surgical instruments contaminated with mad cow and that his neighbor's mother was infected when she took nutritional supplements made from bovine protein—what he calls "mad cow in a pill."

Early on, deep in his grief, Singeltary would introduce himself to scientists in e-mails thus: "In my continued search as to who is responsible for murdering my mom . . . ," and end with "I am the madson of a deadmom who died of madcow." Since then, as his wife, Bonnie, points out, "Terry's calmed down some." From a computer in his living room, Singeltary posts almost daily to CJD and scientific mail lists and message boards to get out the Creutzfeldt Jakobin point of view. With others, he notes that in America there is still no ban on eating those parts of a cow that show the most prion infectivity. Brains, intestines, and mechanically recovered meat—meat that has been blasted off the skeleton of the cow by water pressure and is thus heavy with potentially infectious nerve tissue—are all still for sale. There is no restriction on using bovine protein to make drugs or protein supplements of the sort Terry believes killed his neighbor's mother, either. After the Washington mad cow, the FDA proposed a ban on some of these practices—and then quietly dropped the idea. In the United States it is still legal to feed chicken droppings to cattle, and since chickens are fed cattle protein—some from downer cattle—and prions survive excretion, cattle may in turn be ingesting their own contaminated prions in the chicken feces. (This state of affairs is worrisome enough that McDonald's, the largest user of beef in the country, com-plained in a 2005 letter to the FDA.)

Most relatives of CJD sufferers whom I interviewed agree with Sin-geltary that it was not a sporadic illness that killed their loved ones. They share his two other assumptions as well: first, that all or nearly all CJD in America is caused by infection; second, that the federal govern-ment is hiding this fact from the public. A surprising number of main-stream scientists also doubt the existence of sporadic CJD—among them protein experts, epidemiologists, and neurologists. Their objec-tion is that sporadic CJD is an unnecessary idea. If a disease is known to spread by infection, why assume that some people also get it by chance? Why not find the infectious source in their cases as well? They see theoretical gaps in the idea of sporadic CJD theory too. For one thing, it is strange, if sporadic CJD comes about as a result of the body's declining ability as it ages to manufacture proteins correctly, the chance of getting sporadic CJD goes down at around seventy years of age. And they point out the suspicious coincidence that there has never been a case of sporadic scrapie or BSE in Australia and New Zealand, two countries that are also free of the infectious forms of the disease in native-born animals. Researchers see plenty of possible al-ternative infectious origins for these "sporadic" CJD occurrences, from infected beef, to contamination from hospital instruments, to blood transfusions from people with undiagnosed prion disease (sev-eral such cases recently emerged in Britain), to protein supplement pills, to the bovine protein casing used in many pharmaceuticals, to cosmetics made with cattle byproducts. Peter Crino, Carrie Mahan's neurologist at the University of Pennsylvania Medical Center, is among the sporadic CJD doubters, as are Carleton Gajdusek and David Asher, a former student of Gajdusek's who heads the FDA unit in charge of protecting the country's blood supply.

Among the public, the confusing nomenclature for prion diseases also feeds the doubt. How many people can keep straight the difference among genetic CJD (the kind you are born with a mutation for), sporadic CJD (the kind that happens by chance), and variant CJD (the kind that comes from infection)? I ran into people all the time as I wrote this book who told me "my mother's cousin died of mad cow" or "I have a friend whose aunt died of mad cow." Every time it turned out the relative was diagnosed with sporadic CJD, not the infectious kind, but the family remained skeptical: the victim ate a lot of meat or spent a week in England in the 1980s.

If CJD were not such a brutal death, perhaps the idea of sporadic CJD would not elicit so much resistance. But the relatives of the dead cry out, as sixteen-year-old Vicky Rimmer's grandmother Beryl did, "Why Vicky? A child so healthy? . . . If she had been a sickly child for years, I would have understood." "People just don't die like this without reason," Terry Singeltary told me in a similar vein. Some CJD sufferers become horribly itchy, as if they have scrapie. They scream and howl as if they were being pursued by demons. They see imaginary men climbing into their hospital rooms. Clare Tomkins thought she saw a stick insect on her arm and Carrie Mahan heard the same song in her head over and over. As the relative of one variant CJD sufferer said in 1995: "I couldn't see bloody Satan turn round and say: 'Here, I've invented this one.' "

There is another prion disease in America, chronic wasting disease. If mad cow is the story of disease created in pursuit of profit, CWD is the story of disease created in the pursuit of status. The disease afflicts elk and deer and has now been found in animal populations in half a dozen states and in Canada and South Korea. The symptoms of chronic wasting disease are similar to those of other prion diseases—the animal first sweats and urinates excessively, then begins to lose weight, becomes unstable on its legs, and finally collapses. Mad cow has only been confirmed in a handful of cases in America; by contrast, we know that chronic wasting disease has almost certainly already killed thousands of deer.

A prion plague should not be possible among ruminants in the wild. Deer are not cannibals, as the cows that spread BSE were forced to be; and, because deer and elk are not domesticated, they do not have enough contact with one another to spread a prion infection the way sheep are thought to spread scrapie. But deer do not live as they used to live, humans having once again brought their ambitions to bear on the natural course of things.

The first recorded cases of chronic wasting disease came from Colorado, in the late 1970s. There, a decade before, a young biologist named Gene Schoonveld was at work for the state's division of wildlife in Fort Collins on an experiment meant to help deer survive the winter. This was a new goal in the field. Starvation is one way nature adjusts the deer population to the available food supply. People did not usually see this process, but in the 1950s and 1960s Colorado became more densely settled, reducing forested areas and forcing deer to look longer and harder for food. At the same time, the state enacted conservation laws, limiting when and where hunters could shoot. Soon emaciated deer began wandering onto the lawns and through suburban streets looking for a meal. People began to feed them, only to find that they died anyway. They would drop dead by haystacks, along highways, and in flower beds.

Schoonveld wanted to answer the mystery of why, so he put a group of starving deer in pens at the Colorado State University animal facility. He cut windows in their stomachs to see what went on inside, and then he began to feed them. It turned out that when deer are poorly fed, their ability to absorb nutrients diminishes, because the microorganisms in their stomachs die off. You can give them all the food you want and they won't be able to digest it. They will starve anyway.

During his study, Schoonveld also kept extra deer in a pen next to the starving ones, deer that he hoped would foal and give him docile reserve animals. That pen also held a few sheep that Schoonveld had borrowed from the university for comparative nutritional studies. There is not universal agreement on whether the sheep were infected (many people involved have since died), but Schoonveld says—and some others have confirmed—that there was scrapie in the university's flocks. The scrapie may then have passed from sheep to deer in the same pens.

At first, Schoonveld says he did not notice anything odd—his deer were starving despite his feeding them, as he expected. The surprising part, though, was what was going on with the replacement deer in the holding pen. They had become bedraggled, stumbling, trembling, salivating a lot and losing weight.

What was killing the deer in the holding pens? It couldn't be their food, which was excellent and nutritious. Schoonveld concluded his experiment, wrote it up, leaving out the mystery of the backup deer, and moved on. He did not think twice when Colorado wildlife personnel, in accordance with the department's guidelines, removed the surviving wild deer and released them back into the Rockies.

Ten years later, in 1977, a Colorado State University veterinary graduate student was surprised to find spongiform encephalopathy in the brains of some deer from local pens that she had been given to autopsy. State wildlife officials then began to look around to see how widespread the new scrapie-like disease was. The ten years since Schoonveld's experiments (assuming his deer were the first carriers of the infection) had given CWD a long time to spread. It was now in the eastern part of Colorado and Wyoming in captive herds and soon it was clear it had begun to affect elk too. Eventually it was on the western side of the Rockies, in 2001 it was found in Nebraska, and by 2002 it had crossed the Mississippi and gotten as far as Wisconsin. The disease was even found in 2005 in a captive deer herd in New York State—the deer had been slaughtered and served at a banquet for 350 hunting enthusiasts. At the end of 2005, the first case in a wild moose was reported.

Researchers still don't know a great deal about CWD, but they think the way it spreads more closely resembles scrapie than BSE—that is, contact is crucial. The more deer-to-deer contact, the more infected deer—and deer populations are exploding in America. Schoonveld, now in his early sixties, blames himself for the outbreak. "I fed them. I handled them. I ate them. I gave them to my children to eat," he says. "If anyone should be dead from this disease, it's me." But while Schoonveld might have started CWD—and that will be hard to prove—the disease would not have gotten far without help from a lot of other people along the way.

Deer don't travel a thousand miles in a year on their own. But it turns out that they didn't have to, because people were moving them around the country, inadvertently helping along this new prion disease. Deer farms exist for the purpose of growing deer bigger and with larger antlers than exist in the wild. Since hunters are willing to pay tens of thousands of dollars for the chance to shoot such deer, a deer farm will ship a deer anywhere the hunter wants to go to kill it. Not all farmed deer are shot, though: some escape and breed, and some of those that did also passed on the disease.

But neither the deer that nature had provided nor the deer that farms had shipped satisfied the appetite for the perfect trophy deer. Here another, complementary possible explanation kicks in to explain the fast spread of CWD in recent years. In the world of deer hunting, prize antlers are the goal. The ideal is the ten-point buck, a deer whose rack is so developed it forks into ten branches. Genes affect horn size, but nutrition plays a role too. Could one feed bucks into the trophy books? The idea first gained currency in the late 1960s, when hunting enthusiasts in Texas began a program called "Quality Deer Management," that quickly caught on elsewhere. "Antlers—there is something magical and mystical about deer antlers" one QDM website notes. The protein to make those antlers grow came in the form of feed cakes that hunters could leave wherever deer liked to graze: the deer would eat the cakes and grow more impressive antlers. The project worked: targeted feeding increased the number of prize bucks tenfold. The deer kept getting bigger and bigger and hunters' dens filled with trophies.

The hunters were not aware—any more than the farmers in Britain had been—that the cake they were putting out contained protein from downed animals, including sheep. If scrapie was in the cake—as is likely—the deer would have been exposed to it. The deer gathered in groups for the cakes, and the increased contact among the deer further spread the disease.

In 2002, wildlife officials found CWD in deer near Mount Horeb, Wisconsin, in an area where hunters had been leaving out protein cakes for some years. "We'd come from dairy farming families," one woman who belonged to a local Quality Deer Management group told the Madison paper *The Capital Times,* "so we took our cues for improving the herd from that background." I visited Mount Horeb that fall as it was trying to eradicate the disease. The town has a timeless quality to it: the quiet main street, with its malt shop, is lined with enormous carved wooden trolls in homage to the town's Scandinavian roots. Nearby, Wisconsin's Department of Natural Resources was at work. The DNR was planning to kill every deer in a roughly four-hundred-square-mile area—approximately 25,000 of them. Then it was going to import fresh animals and so save the state's huge deer-hunting business. The plan was modeled on farmers' scrapie-control efforts: eliminate and repopulate.

In many states, the state would have had to call out the National

Guard for such an onslaught, but hunting is a passion in Wisconsin. Hunters shoot 450,000 deer every year, more than in any other state. "I'm . . . looking for ardent hunters to help us, unless fear or their wives keep them away," one DNR official told a Milwaukee magazine. The state extended the normal hunting season and waived the usual limit of one buck per hunter, and the hunters came out in force.

The weekend I was there, deer were everywhere too. They were in every pasture and along every road. You'd turn a corner and a dozen deer would lift their heads: some already had the beginnings of their russet winter coats. I did not see any obviously sick deer—you can count the ribs on a deer with advanced CWD. In the evening, I went to the CWD control station in the woods. I could smell it before I could see it. Hunters were supposed to bring their kills here, where DNR employees and volunteers, wearing bright orange hats that said "Chronic Wasting Disease Response Team," would saw the heads off and place them in coolers to be sent for testing. The hunter had the option of taking the carcass with him to await a clean bill of health or leaving it behind. Ninety percent chose the latter, and the night I was in the field the abandoned bodies were piling up in a tractor-trailer truck, their coats fading, their tongues hanging out. Flies were inescapable; and the participants clearly were not enjoying themselves. "This is hunting for slob hunters," one said. The officials poured a steady supply of a bleach-based disinfectant on the surfaces the deer carcasses had lain on to clean them, believing it would remove all the prion infectivity. In fact, there's dispute over this technique—there's not much that kills a prion for sure.

The next day I went to a University of Wisconsin lab, where veterinary pathology students in head-to-toe protective clothing were extracting the deer's tonsils and their vagus nerve, which runs from the brain into the stomach and is the first site of CWD infection. It was a depressing vista—the heads were gray, the tongues extruded and now blue, and several birds suspected of West Nile virus waited for examination on aluminum tables nearby. It felt like nature was falling apart before our eyes.

The culling established an almost 2 percent infection rate, very high for a disease in the wild. The 2002 hunt did not kill all the deer, and so the eradication program was extended to 2003, then 2004, and continued in 2005. By the third year, 2004, the original target area—reflected in an impressive topographical map at the DNR field head-quarters—had grown from almost 400 square miles to 1,500 square miles to keep up with the spread of the disease. Within the most inten-sively infected zone, the 2004 hunt found an infection rate of 8 percent to 12 percent, a rate that did not change in 2005. Given the DNR's es-timate that without human intervention CWD would infect 40 percent of deer statewide within ten to thirty years, this could be interpreted as meaning that the DNR had fought the disease to a standstill. On the other hand, as one DNR official admitted in 2005: "Eradication is a nice idea, but it's not going to happen." In other words, chronic wast-ing disease is now in Wisconsin to stay.

The key unanswered question about CWD is whether it can be passed to humans the way mad cow can. In 2000, Byron Caughey of the NIH was able to get CWD prions to infect healthy human prion pro-teins in a test tube, but test tubes and real life differ; Caughey says he would not eat venison from an area with CWD, but he also notes the re-assuring molecular differences between CWD prions and human ones. In 2006, a group of researchers found prions in deer muscle meat, meaning that there is at least a potential risk to anyone who eats in-fected venison.

Noting CWD's rapid spread, in 2001, the USDA declared chronic wasting disease a "national emergency." Many European prion re-searchers think it will take more than that to shake America out of its complacency. In 2002, Adriano Aguzzi, an important prion re-searcher in Switzerland, warned Americans that the "threat-from-within" of CWD was being underestimated. "Its horizontal spread among the wild population is exceedingly efficient, and it appears to have reached a prevalence unprecedented even by BSE in the UK at its peak."

Thanks to the USDA's secrecy and sloppiness, Creutzfeldt Jakobins do not need chronic wasting disease to be scared. Whenever there are a lot of CJD cases in a state in a short time, they bring up the possibility of an outbreak of mad cow in humans or variant CJD. There have in recent years been such clusters in Allentown, Pennsylvania; Athens, Georgia; the heartland of South Carolina; Nassau County and Ulster County in New York, and, in late 2005, Idaho. Creutzfeldt Jakobins point out common factors among the sufferers—surgery in the same hospital or meals at the same restaurant, for example—to make the case that an outbreak rather than chance is behind the surprising occurrence of so much CJD in a small area in a short time.

The biggest possible cluster is one associated with the Garden State Race Track, which operated until 2001, in Cherry Hill, New Jersey. If it is ever established that Carrie Mahan had variant CJD—Gambetti's second test also came back negative and her brother has now sent her tissue to England for transmission studies—she will be its first confirmed victim. It was a friend of hers named Janet Skarbek who first identified the pattern of CJD deaths around the racetrack, where Mahan worked. Skarbek is different from Terry Singeltary and most other Creutzfeldt Jakobins in that she defines herself as mainstream, a soccer mom, and a Republican. Her husband is a financial planner; they are people with plenty of reason to trust the system. Janet was not suspicious about Carrie's death in 2000 from CJD. She thought of it as "a tragedy," she says, but nothing more.

Three years later, in June 2003, she happened to be reading a local newspaper. Scanning the obituaries she came across one for a woman named Carol Olive. Olive had also died from CJD—and, like Carrie

Mahan and a hundred or so other people, she had worked at the Garden State Race Track. "That's when I almost fell over," Skarbek remembers: She did a database search and found another CJD victim, John Weber, who lived in Pennsauken, a neighboring town, and had died in 2000. Weber's brother told Skarbek that John held a season pass to the Garden State Race Track and "ate there at least once a week."

As an accountant, Skarbek believed in numbers. She calculated that out of the small group of the track's season pass holders and administrative employees, one person should die of CJD every 909 years, not three in four years. She kept digging and she kept finding people in the area who had died of CJD. In 1997, Jack Schott, a fifty-nine-year-old truck dispatcher, had died of the disease. CJD had also killed a jazz musician named Kenneth Shepherd in 2003, and in the same year, a seventy-one-year-old man, John LaPaglia, Sr. Skarbek began to get tips from friends and families and found two more victims: Walter Z., an IRS accountant, and Alfred P., both of whom died in 1997 from CJD.

Skarbek could connect each of the new victims to the racetrack: Alfred P. had dined there once with a New Jersey congressman. Both Walter Z. and John LaPaglia had been season pass holders. Kenneth Shepherd's wife remembered his eating at the track. Schott went in the early 1990s. "He had the beef," Skarbek said. "His wife had the fish." Carol Olive, her sister said, was "a lover of hamburgers."

Skarbek informed the Centers for Disease Control and the New Jersey Department of Health. She explained that a quick look at a map revealed that four of the victims lived in towns that bordered on Cherry Hill. The total population of these towns was 124,121. Since the natural occurrence of sporadic CJD was supposed to be one person in a million, a population this size should experience a case only once every eight years, she calculated. The CDC and the state health department weren't interested in Skarbek's data. When the first infected cow was found in 2003, Skarbek suspended her accounting practice to devote herself full time to the Garden State Race Track cluster.

One obvious problem with Skarbek's assertions was that the pathologists who had looked at the brains of these supposedly sporadic CJD victims had not seen variant CJD; they had seen sporadic CJD. The two diseases look very different. The sporadic type tends to produce holes in the brain. The variant type is also typically characterized by amyloid plaques, those thick deposits of dead prions in the brain, in addition to holes.

To overcome this difficulty and show a connection among the cases, Skarbek relied on a study by John Collinge, the English prion researcher. Collinge had found in an experiment in 2002 that variant CJD can sometimes look like sporadic CJD in mice with human prion genes. Although what happens in mice cannot necessarily be extrapolated to humans, it was a tantalizing finding. Skarbek was also familiar with the Richard Marsh study from the 1990s that suggested there might be an indigenous strain of BSE in America that didn't look the way mad cow had in Britain. Skarbek believed such a strain was present in the meat served to people who went to the Garden State Race Track; that it had infected them and then the strain had emerged as a form of variant CJD that resembled sporadic CJD. She narrowed down the window of infection to a one-week period between 1988 and 1992.

For Skarbek to be right, there would have to be a strain of mad cow disease in humans in America that was rare enough, or different enough from variant CJD in Britain, to have avoided detection. This is not a scenario American CJD experts find very likely. Ermias Belay, the head of prion surveillance at the CDC, said he thought that if there were a second variant of mad cow in humans, it would have already shown up in Britain, a point with which Collinge himself agrees.

The pattern of infection Skarbek was positing at the Garden State Race Track presented problems, too. The strain of BSE would have to have been present in a single cow or a few cows whose meat was consumed by only the small group of people who ate at a single venue over a short period of time more than a decade ago. And although a tiny amount of BSE prion can cause a fatal infection in cows—a 2005 study showed that a thousandth of a gram would do it—experts in Britain generally believe that repeated consumption of infected proteins plays a role in infecting humans, that the effect is somehow cumulative, because if one bite could do it, the beef the British consumed during the mad cow years would have wiped out most of the island. The idea that a dozen people took the wrong bite of meat at the racetrack doesn't really sound like a prion disease outbreak. It better fits the model of a conventional disease, a salmonella outbreak, for instance, where a discrete group comes into contact with an infectious agent at a particular moment.

In response to Skarbek's agitation and the extensive publicity it received—New Jersey's two U.S. senators called for an investigation—the CDC and the state department of health eventually looked into the cause of death and the autopsy reports of those CJD victims she had found. With the help of Pierluigi Gambetti, the CDC released a report in May 2004. Of the seventeen victims Skarbek brought to their attention, they determined that eleven died of CJD, three had died of other identifiable causes, and the cause of death for the remaining three was not clear. In addition, none of the victims whose genetic makeup could be determined had the methionine-methionine polymorphism that all the variant CJD victims to date in Britain had. This meant they were unlikely to have contracted CJD from infection.

Skarbek was not satisfied: "They're investigating it to disprove it," she told me. In the hopes of getting results that confirm her suspicion, she now encourages families of sufferers not to send tissue samples to establishment researchers like Gambetti but to mavericks, like Frank Bastian, a professor of medicine at Tulane University, who believes that prions are not themselves infectious but accompany an ordinary bacterium that is spread by insects.

Even though she got nowhere with the CDC, Skarbek's quest touched a nerve with the public. She was a middle-class Erin Brock-

ovich, willing to face the risk of a lawsuit from the aggressive beef industry and the ridicule of the USDA and the CDC to declare that mad
cow was already in America. Congress asked her to testify on the risk of
variant CJD in America, and the Japanese consulted with her on their
American beef embargo. A filmmaker is at work on a documentary
about her crusade.

Although she is the most prominent self-appointed mad cow researcher, Skarbek is far from the only one. Wherever a cluster pops up,
someone is there to estimate the odds against it. (The longest odds of
all were in a case reported by Carleton Gajdusek of an American husband and wife who died of supposedly sporadic CJD four and a half
years apart; the odds of this are one in a trillion; Gajdusek says he believes the couple were infected by an unknown route.)

The war cry of the Creutzfeldt Jakobins is the adage "Absence of evidence isn't evidence of absence." This stance invites the amateur into
medicine, since it suggests that no authority is definitive and we all
may have something to contribute to the search for a cause or cure. Of
course, no one should forget that in Britain those who refused to accept the official position were proved to be right, that in fact it was pre-
cisely those scientists and journalists who bucked authority to whom
the British owe their thanks.

The CDC report sidestepped the real question Skarbek was raising
because it had no answer for it: what *would* variant CJD in America
look like? Would it resemble the strain in Britain? What would its molecular signature be? What age group would it strike? And would it
occur in clusters? There is no reason to assume that food would even
have to be the vector for the disease; Gajdusek's deputy C. J. Gibbs,
who handled cases of CJD that came to the NIH's attention, once
noted that all the sporadic CJD victims he had met had been avid gardeners. Plant foods contain bone meal from cow protein, too.

The Creutzfeldt Jakobins are a crowd slowly growing into a movement, because even if the mad cow scare passes, worries about our

food supply will remain. Until a few years ago, postings on the websites run by CJD sufferers' families, such as CJD Watch and CJD Voice, were mostly from people whose relatives had sporadic CJD, wanting contact with others who'd been through the same experience. Over time, as mad cow began to agitate the American psyche, the postings became more political. They began to come from people like Singeltary and Skarbek, who believed, as Singeltary put it, that "mad cow is here, it's killing people and those assholes aren't doing anything about it."

Most recently, people who think they may have variant CJD have begun posting their symptoms. "I have had problems now for more then two and a half years, started positional vertigo, then fever and the fassiculations [*sic*] started all over . . . and I feel its hard to think," an anonymous poster wrote on the CJD Watch website in June 2003. A young man posted in summer 2004 to report his fear that he had caught mad cow, citing "weird spells." "The spells went away," he explained, "but then I got panic attacks where I would just feel like I was flipping out for no reason. Then those went away." His current symptoms were "muscle twitching all over my body (face, limbs, trunk, etc.); several kinds of twitching: small, localized fasciculations just underneath the skin. Difficulty with abstract thought. Poor short term memory. Brain fog. Bad math skills and reduced spelling. Apathy (very little emotion). Myoclonus 2 types (when I try to sleep, it wakes me up) and another that happens when I'm awake. Constant, high-pitched tone in my head. Bad floaters (regular squiggles and bizarre swimming specks). Tremors that usually occur when I use my muscles. Examples: If I scrunch up my nose, my face tremors, if I make a tight fist, my hand shakes. Anytime any muscle tenses up, it tremors."

A Latina woman who thought she had gotten variant CJD from taking a supplement for breast enlargement soon joined him on the message board. The symptoms she reported were similar to his, including panic attacks, myoclonic jerks, and incipient blindness. She was certain she was dying, but, as the young man pointed out to her in 2005, given that she had been on the message board for almost two years by then, "the fact that you're not only alive, but apparently using a computer, walking, etc. means you probably don't have vcjd [variant CJD]." Nothing could dissuade the woman, who kept approaching new doctors in search of a diagnosis. "You seem almost to want to have some form of VCJD," an irritated poster wrote to her in early 2006. "From what I have read it is so immenently clear that you do not that anyone could see it. Whatever you have that is not a serious emotional problem is not VCJD." The poster added, "Psychiatric help. Get some." Yet she in turn was able to castigate a woman who promised that she had cured herself of CJD with Mini Oxygen Therapy. "Quitt offering falses hopes, to people who really are dealing with cjd. Sorry! but this is the reality," she wrote in February 2006. To which the woman who said she'd been cured responded with accidental ambiguity, "I don't believe my information gives false hope—at the moment, what else is there?"

The takeover of the CJD message board list upset the original grieving CJD families—that small group who still believed what the experts told them, that their loved ones just died by chance. One bristled at what she called the "whining from hypochondriacs and wild theories of cover ups from the tin foil hat crowd." But she was ignored. Nothing could stop the Creutzfeldt Jakobins, because in a world where absence of evidence isn't evidence of absence, no one can prove you aren't sick, either.

PART IV

AWAKENINGS?

CHAPTER 15

FOR THE VICTIMS OF FATAL
FAMILIAL INSOMNIA THE VENETO, *present day*

Throughout the 1990s, members of the Italian family with fatal familial insomnia kept dying. In 1993, Pierluigi Gambetti in Cleveland developed a test for the mutation that causes the disease, and, at Lisi and Ignazio's urging, fifty relatives went to Bologna and had their blood drawn. At last something definite was known. But in fact, the knowledge was not airtight. The test returned a considerable percentage of wrong results—as high as 15 percent in the beginning.

Some members of the family refused to take the test, worried that the stressful process would itself bring on the family disease. One such man was cousin Carlo, whose brother Flavio had died of FFI in 1974. After Flavio's death came his brother Terenzio in 1975. Carlo tried to live a quiet life and slip past the age of onset, and at sixty-one he thought he'd succeeded. But one evening in 1996, he came to see his niece Lucia. Lucia had helped raise the children her sister Teresa had left behind and had joined forces with Ignazio and Lisi in trying to find a cure. Lucia had seen a lot of death from FFI by then: her grandfather,

father, two uncles, and Teresa. She knew what it looked like. She could tell from Uncle Carlo's shrunken pupils what his fate would be. She sent him to Ignazio, who sent him to Bologna; Lucia and Carlo's wife accompanied him on the train ride. "I knew. He knew," Lucia says. "Maybe his wife knew." Carlo died shortly after.

Some branches of the family were particularly hard hit, yet, through death after death, they kept their deep faith in God. Sometimes, in fact, the onslaught sent them back to the Church. This was the case for a young man I'll call Arturo. Arturo is intense, with Marianna's flaming-red hair and a forceful urge to question. He lost three uncles to the disease before he was thirty. In his teens he contacted the Bologna neurologist Pietro Cortelli to see if the insomnia he suffered might be a sign of the disease (Cortelli reassured him he was too young). Arturo was determined to break his family's taboo about discussing the disease and to confront it in a modern manner. He even went to the library and pulled out a book on the subject. He saw the fateful misfolded proteins that were killing his family. In 2000, his father began to have trouble sleeping. The family tried to keep him out of Bologna. They had had enough of the institute. Instead they took him to several regional hospitals, where finally the doctors urged them to go to Cortelli and Elio Lugaresi without wasting further time. Eventually he did.

The family had been praying throughout this time, reciting the Rosary every night. Their faith deepened with their suffering. They believed and it gave them strength. As he weakened, Arturo's father told him he was not afraid to die and reminded him to take care of his mother and his sister after he was gone—Arturo would, after all, be the new head of the family. A month later, Arturo's father developed a soaring fever, then fell into a coma and soon after died. The doctors at Bologna hoped to be able to do an autopsy and ship the brain to Pierluigi Gambetti, as it was accustomed to do, but the family, including Arturo, did not want that. Arturo, who until now had been the family goad, had had a change of heart. His father had had a good death in the

Lord. That they had prayed together every night gave him more comfort than the EEGs or the doctors. Arturo looked forward to seeing his father in heaven.

When I spoke to him a week later, his conversion was clear. He no longer wanted to be the family firebrand. His intensity had turned inward in a search for a serenity that would ward off the disease. He became the sacristan of his church and ate only holistic foods. When I asked him if he was going to take the test now to see if he had the mutation that had killed his grandmother, his father, and three uncles, he told me no. The anxiety over the test itself might bring the disease. Besides, what would he do with the information? There wasn't a cure.

What happens to the Italian family in the end depends less on their own actions than on the world's interest in prion diseases, which they cannot control. If lots of people are afraid of getting variant CJD, the family benefits. If fear of prion disease goes the way of the fear of swine flu or Ebola, then they will be orphaned again.

The mad cow years left them better positioned than before, but still a long way from safety. How do you fight a disease that remains so much a mystery? A killer protein whose function when healthy is unknown and whose method of causing cell death is obscure? Not since Pasteur's time have researchers attempted to counter an infection knowing so little about what they are fighting.

The ideal way to defeat a pathogen is to develop an artificial molecule that can bond with it and lock it up. Unfortunately, researchers aren't sure of the shape of the prion. Besides, to develop a drug from scratch takes a decade and costs around $750 million to $1 billion. Researchers designed some of the anti-HIV drugs this way, but millions of people have HIV. By contrast, there are roughly forty known families with FFI in the world. Add to that number the families that have related genetic prion diseases—genetic CJD or Gerstmann-Sträussler-

Scheinker disease—and the number is up to three hundred. Add in all the families who have a member suffering from or who has already died of variant CJD or CJD caused by growth hormone and you are up to five hundred affected families. Five hundred families do not constitute a critical mass in the world of medical research, no matter how spectacular their symptoms or how grievous the governmental error that made some of them sick. When in 1997 the British government called a meeting to discuss cures for variant CJD, representatives of only three pharmaceutical companies showed up: there was simply not enough money in it for them.

So researchers work with existing drugs to try to cure prion disease. There are about a hundred significantly different compounds in use to combat all diseases. Fewer than fifteen of these can cross into the brain, where prions do most of their damage. Lab machines can automatically test variations of these compounds against material infected with prions. If a drug shows promise, the researcher can move right to a human trial—there is no need for laborious proofs that the drug is safe, since it has already been approved for other human diseases. The only question the researcher has to answer is whether it is effective.

The first drug to come down the pipeline this way was quinacrine. During World War II, malaria was a big concern for American troops. The cure—in fact, the first cure for any disease—was quinine, derived from the bark of the cinchona tree. Because the drug was so useful, over the years many governments, organizations, and scientists—the Jesuit order and Baron Liebig among them—tried to corner the supply. At the beginning of World War II, the Japanese occupied most of the Far East, where the cinchona trees grew. In response, American scientists put into wide production a synthetic replacement. American troops took millions of doses of quinacrine, and cases of malaria among them declined to nearly zero.

Quinacrine consists of very small molecules. That was its first attractive quality for prion researchers—it could get through the blood-brain barrier. By 1997, labs were trying compounds derived from quinacrine on test tubes of mouse cells infected with prions. A Japanese researcher named Katsumi Doh-Ura, working with Byron Caughey of the NIH, first published a report that the drug could reduce infectivity in 2000, but as usual Prusiner's lab in San Francisco, which came out with similar findings a year later, got the credit.

In the summer of 2001, an Englishman named Stephen Forber was searching the Internet for a cure for his twenty-year-old daughter, Rachel, one of the hundred or so Britons who had been diagnosed with variant CJD by that time. Forber contacted Stephen Dealler, the English microbiologist who had warned early on that mad cow would cross to humans. After Dealler's fears had come true, he began to push for a cure.

Dealler had heard that Prusiner's lab was having some luck with quinacrine, so when Forber contacted him, he put him in touch with Prusiner's researchers and they agreed to give Rachel quinacrine. The drug was safe at the doses necessary to prevent malaria, but those doses were too low to block a prion disease. Still, Prusiner had been promising a cure for a long time and the initial results from quinacrine— admittedly just in mouse cells—had been very encouraging. His team started Rachel on the drug. What happened next was miraculous: Rachel got better. She had arrived in San Francisco in June unable to walk or talk or recognize what was going on around her. Four weeks after that, she was nearly herself.

The British government had been stalling on funding prion cure research, but Rachel's apparent recovery prompted it to put up £200,000 for further quinacrine trials. For Prusiner, it was sweet revenge. The government that kept him out of the mad cow drama was now beginning to understand what it had missed. Three years before, he had predicted that he could cure CJD in five years, and here he was two years ahead of schedule. Then things fell apart.

Quinacrine at high doses causes sterility, shaking, and liver damage. That was why, as soon as the military could replace quinacrine with another synthetic cure for malaria, it did. Rachel Forber was getting a very high dose of quinacrine: in the hospital, she was so yellow from liver damage that doctors called her "the lemon princess." After her discharge, her liver began to fail. She had to stop the pills. As the quinacrine left her system, her symptoms returned. She went downhill quickly, dying in December 2001, six months after her diagnosis. By now, more than three hundred prion disease sufferers have tried quinacrine and, according to Graham Steel, the head of the CJD Alliance in the United Kingdom, "they're all dead."

Prusiner's many enemies blamed the Forber fiasco on him. His lab, though, considered the treatment a success. According to them, postmortem studies of Rachel's cells showed a great decline in prion infectivity. And what had been the alternative? "When you have someone with a fatal illness, then anything is okay," said Fred Cohen, a biochemist who worked closely with Prusiner to treat Rachel. He is now trying to make a less toxic variation of quinacrine.

After Forber's death, the families of most CJD sufferers put their faith in a different drug, pentosan. Derived from beechwood, pentosan is usually prescribed for infections of the lining of the bladder. In 1984, Alan Dickinson, then the irascible head of the Neuropathogenesis Unit in Edinburgh, first tried it on mice infected with scrapie. He found that even a very low dose of pentosan delayed the onset of the disease. Over the years, various researchers tried pentosan on rats, hamsters, and dogs with similar success. Dickinson considered giving it to humans too, but he never did—he was worried about side effects. Pentosan is a blood thinner and too high a dose can cause seizures.

In time, another father with a sick child found his way to Stephen Dealler. Donald Simms had read about pentosan on the Web. His twenty-two-year-old son Jonathan, a former star soccer player, was dying of variant CJD in Belfast. Could Dealler help Jonathan get pentosan? Dealler explained that the problem with the drug was that it was too large to cross the blood-brain barrier. It might help someone who had just been infected by prions, before the prions had had a chance to make their way into the central nervous system, but Jonathan's was not a new infection.

Dealler also told Simms that no one in Britain was actively pursuing pentosan, but Simms, a gruff, heavy-smoking contractor who is built like a rugby player, was not easily deterred. By chance, Doh-ura, the Japanese researcher who first tested quinacrine on prions, was coming to Scotland. Don Simms found him by calling ninety hotels in Edinburgh. The researcher told him what he hoped to hear: Pentosan might be able to slow down or stop the prion infection.

The problem of how to get pentosan into Jonathan's brain was not insurmountable, either. In recent years researchers had learned how to put shunts through the skull to deliver cancer drugs. Simms was able to find a neurosurgeon willing to carry out a similar procedure on Jonathan. Simms's next problem was getting the British government to allow it. The Rachel Forber episode had traumatized the English medical establishment. There was worry that the young victims of variant CJD were at risk of being betrayed twice—once by the government, the second time by their own parents. Simms sued and in 2003 won his son the right to the treatment. Astonishingly, the boy had survived the seventeen-month delay.

Jonathan's treatment has been more successful than Rachel Forber's. Pentosan is effective because the molecule binds to a site necessary for prion proteins to convert to malignant prions. It works the way putting a dummy key into a lock prevents another key from turning the mechanism. Doctors gave Jonathan less than a year to live after his initial diagnosis in 2001. Yet he is still alive as this book goes to press, five years later, the longest-living prion disease sufferer known. He is, though, hardly well. If Rachel Forber's story was one of improbable recovery followed by precipitous decline Jonathan Simms's is of staving off death, perhaps even making tiny steps toward health. His blood pressure is lower, he has regained some of the weight he lost, and his ability to swallow and to sleep has returned. A year after his treatment started, he heard his favorite soccer team was playing, pointed to the TV and said the word "On"—or so it was reported in 2004. Jonathan can look at people again, but he can't roll over in bed or feed himself and likely never will be able to. Scans have shown that his brain is continuing to atrophy, though the progress he seems to be making would suggest the opposite. "Johnny's stable," Donald told me when I saw him at a CJD family conference in 2005, "my boy is stable."

Inevitably, the news of Jonathan Simms's success reached America. The first American to be given pentosan was James Alford. In 2002, when Alford was a twenty-four-year-old Special Forces soldier serving in Iraq, he suddenly started falling apart. He seemed confused and inattentive; he went AWOL. The army suspected him of malingering. In 2003, it demoted Alford from staff sergeant and told him to carry a pen and paper with him to write down orders. The army was on the point of court-martialing Alford for insubordination when a military doctor examined him and diagnosed CJD. Alford was given a medical discharge and in April 2003 allowed to go home to die. Instead, thanks to Terry Singeltary's efforts at getting the word out, Alford became a cause célèbre. When *The O'Reilly Factor* featured his story, the show's resident military commentator called Alford's treatment "the worst case of abuse of a soldier I've seen in thirty years."

Alford believed he was a war casualty. He told others that a banquet he and other soldiers attended while on a covert mission in Oman in 2001 was not the warm welcome it seemed—someone deliberately served a scrapie-infected sheep to the Americans. Alford's hypothesis strikes prion researchers as fanciful, because scrapie has never been shown to be contagious to humans. "We shot monkeys full of scrapie in my lab and nothing happened," Carleton Gajdusek told me when I told him Alford's story. "They're still the monkeys that are there today." All the same, the army, under media pressure, reinstated Alford at full pay and began treating him as if he were a soldier who had caught a disease or taken a bullet in a war. The army also helped Alford get access to pentosan, but the results have not been what they were for Jonathan Simms. Every month Alford's family drives him to a hospital near his home in Karnack, Texas, where doctors mix a few drops of the drug into saline fluid and funnel it through a shunt into his head. When Alford began his treatment in March 2004, he was surviving on fluids. He did not respond to voices. He has not recovered any lost ground—his decline has continued and he is nearly comatose now—still alive, but barely. Stephen Dealler thinks the difference between Alford's response and Jonathan Simms's may be that Simms simultaneously received high doses of Vitamin E, but that remains to be proved. By early 2006, there were about thirty patients with variant or sporadic CJD taking pentosan around the world with all but one still living. The outlook for inherited prion disease victims is not as promising. In 2005, an American woman with an inherited form of GSS who had begun to show symptoms contacted Donald Simms, learned about pentosan, and began treatment. She died at the end of the year, one of three GSS patients to try the drug without much success, suggesting that the virulence of inherited prion diseases is greater than that of sporadic or infectious kinds.

The Italian family watches all this activity. Ignazio reads English well and checks the CJD websites for updates, but neither he nor Lisi nor anyone else in the family is a Donald Simms or a Stephen Forber, willing to go to any length for a cure. Nearly every month there is news about a new drug that blocks prion malformation, but it is always in cell cultures or maybe mice, never people. The developments both excite them and increase their desire to stay on the sidelines. They have seen experts who have sent them to other experts, who have only delivered more expertise. Living with FFI has made them tired. And wary. They know that for all that has been learned about their disease, deliverance is still a long way off.

At the first family reunion in 2001, the talk was of America. The family wanted to have a foundation there. "America," they said, "is where the money and the research are." *Lo zio d'America,* the rich emigrant uncle, is a stock figure in Italians' minds, this family's as well. America had saved Italy many times. America could save Italy again. And in America, some reasoned at the reunion, the family would also be anonymous. They could have both the privacy and the money.

But then they thought about it some more. Prusiner loves prions more than people, they told me. And the prospect of pentosan filled them with horror. Having, as USCF chemist Fred Cohen puts it, "a bolt put in your head" so a technician can "squirt something into your brain" is a high price to pay for a few more years of life.

The family knows that it has value to researchers. People with prion diseases are not easy to come by; large families with a hereditary prion disease even rarer. I was once in Pierluigi Gambetti's office in Cleveland and heard him talking on the phone about some tissue he was expecting. His end of the conversation, in his careful, accented English, went like this: "Do you have a way to keep it frozen? . . . Do you know if it will last un-teel tom-or-row? . . . You have a refrigerator or freeeez-er? Can you add dry ice? . . . We can't get Fed-er-al Ex-press after six pee-em. There is no way to get in. . . . Well, see if it fits in the freeeez-er."

And FFI is a disease of sleeplessness in an era when insomnia affects about 10 percent of the Western world, or some one hundred twenty million people. "If I were the director of the NIH, I would pour money into FFI research," William Dement, the founder of sleep medicine, told me. "You might get a cure for insomnia. At the very least we could make our sleeping pills infinitely safer and more practical." Still the family evaluates its options cautiously, shadowboxing with its past. Recently it teamed up with a prestigious institute for protein research in Milan. The difficult goal of the alliance will be to find a drug that can turn off prion production in skin cells and then get it to do the same thing in the brain.

In the meantime, to raise money and to reach out to other sufferers of FFI, the family launched a website for their association (www.afiff .org/). Its home page features a drawing of Hypnos, the Greek god of sleep, above an inert man. A ticker on the margin of the page scrolls through the latest prion disease research and therapies from around the world. Hypnos looks close enough to it that if he were to just put down his useless trumpet and reach a long arm out, he could pluck a cure that would finally make the figure beneath him wake.

In early 2003, another member of the Italian family got sick. Vittorino lived at the southern end of the Venetian lagoon. He was from a distant branch of the family; its point of intersection with Lisi's branch is so remote that until Ignazio received a call from Vittorino's two daughters, he did not know it existed. The daughters, Maria and Roberta, had seen a recent article on the new fatal familial insomnia association in an Italian newspaper and they wanted to know if the disease their father had might, in fact, be FFI. Vittorino had already been to three hospitals, Sottomarina—where he had been diagnosed as alcoholic—Piove, and Padua, whose neurologists had long since forgotten the mystery of Assunta and Pierina. Ignazio explained the condition to Maria and Roberta and tests given to Vittorino confirmed he had the disease. Before this time, no one in his family had ever heard of FFI.

Vittorino turned out to be a direct descendant of Giuseppe, whose fourteen-year-old son, Costante, was the first certain victim of the disease, in 1828. Maria and Roberta's grandmother and great-grandmother both died of the disease, which their older relatives long referred to as the family curse. No one had ever been willing to talk to the sisters about it.

When, shortly after Vittorino's death, I met Roberta and Maria—

modern, cultured Italians, with stylish hair and eyewear—they were still awestruck by what they had seen. Vittorino, an athletic man, had been reduced to a wraith in months. In the grip of the disease, he mimed happily fishing in the Adriatic. The death itself was terrible to see—the myoclonic jerks, the stupor, the gasping for breath—and yet they were grateful that they were not alone in their suffering, that dozens of distant relatives had been wrestling with the same disease for centuries and that there was even a writer interested in the subject. They told me that after their father died, they made sure that his body was available to researchers. They talked about what had happened with friends. And then they did something else no member of the family had ever done before in two centuries. They placed an offering jar outside the church where the funeral mass was said, with the words "For the victims of fatal familial insomnia" on it for everyone to see.

AFTERWORD: A NOTE ON THE AUTHOR

*I am quite familiar with your disease and hope that our work
will stimulate a cure some day.*

—STANLEY PRUSINER
in a note to the author

By the time I finished researching *The Family That Couldn't
Sleep* I had come to feel an enormous distance between the Italian family with its two-century-long burden and my own situation. I believed
the suffering of those who had FFI—possibly the worst disease in the
world—was unique and must be respected by others. At the beginning
of my research, I had thought that we were truly joined by the fact that
we were both sick and both our diseases involved misfolded proteins,
but by the end that link seemed trivial. They had a fatal, rapid neurodegenerative prion disease. I had a nonfatal, nonprion, slowly progres-
sive, neuromuscular disease. I was, as the young man had said at the
2001 reunion of the Italian family, *un curioso,* at best a thoughtful onlooker, at worst a gawker. Not one of them.

But one day while I was working on this book, I got the correspondence quoted at the head of this chapter. Prusiner was linking us

again—me, the Italian family, CJD sufferers, Huntington's disease and Alzheimer's syndrome sufferers—as in my mind we had been linked when I began.

The connection works this way: the syndrome I have is closely related to spinal muscular atrophy (SMA) and Charcot-Marie-Tooth disease (CMT), two neuromuscular diseases that are like slowed-down versions of amyotrophic lateral sclerosis (ALS, or Lou Gehrig's disease). These diseases are one step further removed from prions than are neurodegenerative disorders such as Huntington's disease and Alzheimer's, which produce amyloid plaque. SMA, CMT, and ALS are neither prion diseases nor amyloid plaque diseases, but they are protein misfolding diseases.

Beyond that, very little about the diseases mine resembles is clear. Take CMT. It is a hodgepodge of some three dozen varied conditions spread out on half a dozen chromosomes. The severity of the different subtypes of CMT varies a great deal. Some people with the syndrome never know it; others need wheelchairs in childhood. I first noticed something was wrong in my late twenties. My left foot had begun to drag. Then one day I felt the ground shifting. In a moment, balancing had become a conscious act. After that, I couldn't simply walk; I walked and balanced. I shook hands and balanced. I talked and balanced. It was as if I were always standing on a water bed. As the disease progressed, a neurologist prescribed me plastic braces, which were hard to put on because my hands had also weakened.

What had happened in my body was that my longest nerves, the ones going from the base of the spine all the way down to my feet and up to my arms, were malfunctioning. They had lost the ability to communicate with the corresponding muscles, a loss that in turn made my legs and arms atrophy. On the molecular level, a mutation in one of my genes had changed the structure or the quantity of proteins needed for my nerves to successfully send electrical signals to my muscles. Nerve electricity conduction involves hundreds of different proteins: proteins to carry the current, proteins to insulate the nerve, proteins to convey electricity efficiently, proteins to repair faulty proteins.

No one knows which mutation I have or on which gene it lies, but the syndrome whose clinical manifestation is most like mine is a form of CMT caused by a mutation on a gene on Chromosome 21. The gene produces a protein called the neurofilament light protein, or NFL. NFLs self-assemble into filaments or wires within the axon, the long stringy part of the nerve. When things go right, the NFLs are very precise, assembling into long tubes that help other molecules go up and down the axon. When Shuguang Zhang of MIT dreams, he dreams of a man-made, self-assembling molecule as nimble as the NFL. But if the NFL gene has a mutation, the protein loses its rigidity and cannot form tubes. The change blocks the traffic in the molecules that help the nerve impulses travel. So my nerves are defective not because there is anything wrong with them but because the scaffolding that holds them together is malformed. The problem is not the telephone wires but the poles.

There are two ways prion research might show the path to fixing this defect. Prion researchers are protein structure experts. They could focus on the error in the NFL protein structure as it was being created and substitute a replacement amino acid that would improve the protein's functioning. Or they could insert a helper protein in my nerve cells that would compensate for the defect in my NFLs and restore their rigidity. You would need decades with either approach before you could predict success or failure, but the knowledge and technology are in place to begin the lab work now—indeed, parallel approaches are being tried in neurodegenerative and prion diseases.

In the event, Prusiner's note turned out to be an overstatement, as a quick clarification from his assistant explained: "What he meant by that statement," the assistant wrote, "was that CMT shares some characteristics with prion disease, which might in turn benefit research on CMT, but he didn't mean to imply that we were working on CMT.

Unfortunately, Dr. Prusiner doesn't know anyone who is working on CMT."

Even if Prusiner had had a magic pill for me, I don't know that I would have taken it. He makes a lot of promises that don't work out (think of the poor "Lemon Princess"). Besides, being sick is a habit, and pursuing a cure disrupts that habit—it can always make you sicker, or at least make you feel sicker, as the Italian family has long known. Not that I'm not tempted by the publicity, the purpose, the celebrity, the affirmation of life that searching for a cure conveys. If my disease someday gets swept up in some *other* brilliant egotistical scientist's quest for a Nobel in the protein disease field, I might say Yes, use me. I know it takes a lot of noise to enable a sick person to live again in what the French doctor René Leriche called "the silence of the organs."

Anyone with a genetic disease also has a responsibility to think about the future. I have two little children. The chances are 50–50 that either will get my mysterious ailment. I watch my son's steps and see that his left foot turns inward—am I seeing the first sign of the disease in him? But then he outgrows it, and I relax. My daughter is learning to crawl late—is that meaningful? But then I remember that I may not have an inherited disease at all. All the genetic tests I have taken have come out negative. No one in my family has similar symptoms. Rather than an unidentified genetic disease, I may have an unidentified sporadic disease—except that I don't really believe in sporadic sickness. The chemicals I was exposed to as a child, the vaccines, the X rays of my teeth, the cans of tuna with their nanograms of mercury: something made me ill, I believe. Why else were all these neuromuscular diseases rare until forty years ago?

So I am a Creutzfeldt Jakobin too, if only up to a point. Charcot, the great French neurologist for whom CMT is named, used to march down the halls of his clinic at the Salpêtrière, the huge Parisian charity ward and hospital where he first identified the disease, and when he saw a sufferer, he would exclaim, "What have we done, O Zeus! To deserve this destiny? Our fathers were wanting, but we, what have we done?" My answer to Charcot's question is "Nothing." We are by nature sick animals and the fabulously long, healthy lives many of us are living today are unnatural, "in opposition," as Richard Parkinson warned in 1810, "to their creator." There is no reason why I should have been singled out for a moderately different version of a familiar (in both senses) neuromuscular disease but also no reason why not.

My Padua is Columbia Presbyterian Medical Center, on top of a windy hill in the northern part of Manhattan, and one morning sometime in the 1990s—but it could be the 2000s or the 2010s, and it could be Montefiore or Baylor or Yale—I am standing in my underpants in front of a neurologist, his attentive students all around. The scene is as it has ever been since Charcot's time—the great doctor with his acolytes. Even the exam has changed little since then. My arms are out. The neurologist wants me to push up while he pushes down. I push up. He wants me to push down while he pushes up. I push down. He wants me to make a circle of my index finger and my thumb. He breaks my grip with his hand. He wants me to close my eyes. He pries them open. He wants me to shut my mouth. He can't open it with his hands. The students watch.

He asks me to sit with my legs out and I do. He pushes down on them. I push up. We push on each other. He is sweating. He stoops and pushes down against my feet and they fold downward like limp petals. He pushes up on my feet and they go up like gates. Even though he never looks me in the eye, I can tell he enjoys this moment.

He takes out a safety pin, opens it, and pricks the bottom of my foot. Sharp, I say. He touches it with the dull part. Dull, I say. (These are my two choices.) He pricks my big toe. Sharp. He grabs a toe and moves it upward. Up, I say. He takes a toe and moves it down. Down. He takes a toe and starts to move it up but then moves it down. Down. I smell my own sweat.

I watch his finger go from right to left and left to right. He snaps the finger in my ear for some reason. He takes a tuning fork from the pocket of his white coat and puts the butt on my foot until it stops vibrating. "Now," I say. He taps my knees and ankles with a rubber-tipped hammer. I want to say to him: "Ankle reflexes diminished, knee reflexes normal," but I don't. Part of the discipline of neurology as Charcot perfected it is that the neurologist must see the disease for himself or herself. He must never trust anyone or anything else. Charcot was a disciple of positivism, a faith aggressive in its humility. Positivism emphasized what you could see, not what you could imagine to be true. In medicine, you could describe how a person dragged his leg, how his muscles seemed weak. You could name the disease "leg-dragging syndrome" or "muscular atrophy," but you could not speculate on whether it was caused by inheritance, an accident, or a previous disease. Positivism tamped down speculation and promoted rigor and classification. Its refusal to explore, now so brutal, felt modern.

"Let someone say of a doctor that he really knows his physiology or anatomy, or that he is dynamic," Charcot once said. "These are not compliments; but when you say he is an observer, a man who knows how to see, this is the greatest compliment you can make." Through positivism, Charcot proposed to do for science what photography had done for painting: replace metaphysical notions with truth. So, like the photographer, the neurologist had to do his work without pity. Charcot once hired a maid with disseminated sclerosis and watched her deteriorate from year to year, enduring what Freud, his student, called "a small fortune in broken plates and platters," until he admitted her to the Salpêtrière, so he could observe her, and after her death, claim her body and make a diagnosis.

Likewise the neurologist in front of me now does not want to hear my observations about my body. He wants to keep pushing on my arms and legs like levers on a flawed machine. The clinician's associate notes the results by decorating a stick figure on a pad of paper with numbers from 1 to 5. I get 4+s and 4−s after our stylized wrestling match, 3+s on the feet. "The patient does not fully bury his eyelashes," he writes—the muscles in my face are weakening. The patient is aware of this, knows he can no longer wink with his left eye. The patient has a V-shaped facies, foot drop, steppage gait, stork legs, and—this sounds particularly menacing—a terminal tremor. He lacks dorsiflexion and his feet are everted.

Some doctors say that neurology attracts the unusually shy or nerdy, medical students more comfortable interpreting the results of a patient's EMG or MRI than talking to him or her about what he or she is experiencing. But I believe the reason no one looks you in the eye during a neurology exam is shame—the neurologist's shame. The fact is that the neurologist can diagnose you but he can't cure you. For him, it is still 1860. Almost 150 years later, he still has nothing more to offer than the accuracy of the clinical gaze. Such impotence touched even Charcot. At the height of his fame, his lectures drew medical students to Paris from all over the world, Freud, Babinski, and La Tourette among them. One day at the Salpêtrière in 1888, Charcot examined a man with a severe neurodegenerative disease. The patient had first noticed a problem sixteen months before. His mind worked fine, but he could no longer speak. He drooled so badly he had to keep a handkerchief with him. His reflexes were exaggerated. Spasmodic jerks rippled under his skin like tiny fish. Charcot took his audience through a tour of this body in disarray and gave his diagnosis, amyotrophic lateral sclerosis—now commonly called Lou Gehrig's disease in the United States, but in Europe known as Charcot's disease. This condition, Charcot boasted, "is one of the most completely understood . . . in the realm of clinical medicine." It was he after all who had done much of the understanding. The exam done, Charcot spoke to the patient for the first time: "My friend, you can leave the room now and you will be told in a minute what you should do in order to get well." The patient's son walked him out. When they were gone, Charcot turned to his fellow doctors and said in a stage whisper, "Now, gentlemen, that the patient is no longer here, we can and must speak amongst ourselves in total frankness. The prognosis is deplorable." Charcot gave the man a few months to live, "perhaps a year at the most."

After my exam, the neurologist invites me to get dressed and come into his office, where his subordinates are already sitting or hovering. He tells me I have a variation of CMT—or SMA. "Or the same disease with a different name," I joke. He doesn't smile. Charcot never did, either. When I ask whether CMT is worse than SMA or SMA worse than CMT, the neurologist always tells me the one I don't have is worse. I am lucky.

My prognosis is not deplorable, just chronic. I walk, I go: the thing happens. I wear braces on my legs. For therapy, I use a small electrical transformer that stimulates my atrophied muscles, a technique with which Charcot experimented. "We know by experience that the electric spark acts most favorably on the nutrition of the muscles," he wrote. I take a powdered amino acid supplement called creatine, an invention of Baron von Liebig. I am now used to my situation. Compared to anyone with a prion disease, I am lucky, indeed, to have the luxury of time enough to get used to anything. When I leave, the neurologist suggests I come back in a year or two. Sometimes I do. Sometimes I don't. Sometimes I go to another doctor instead, to see if something more can be found out. Absence of evidence isn't evidence of absence, after all. Someone somewhere someday will have a cure—or at least a name—for whatever it is that I have.

ACKNOWLEDGMENTS

An enormous, boundless, heartfelt thank you to Ignazio and Elisabetta, to Elisabetta's cousin Lucia and the other members of the Italian family whose story is told in these pages. May this book be a step in vanquishing FFI!

Without the help of two people this book would have taken even longer to be born: Walker Jackson of the Whitehead Institute at MIT, whose deep knowledge of the prion field and gift for explaining it to the nonspecialist strikes me as unique; and Jennifer Harbster, science research librarian at the Library of Congress, whose uncanny knack for finding any book, journal, or newspaper article, no matter how obscure, in that vast collection, ought to win her an award.

In addition, I wish to thank Pierluigi Gambetti, head of the National Prion Disease Pathology Surveillance Center at Case Western Reserve, for his generous help and scientific advice; Howard Kiernan of Columbia Presbyterian Medical Center for his help (and efforts to diagnose my condition); James Lupski of Baylor College of Medicine for sharing his expertise on Charcot-Marie-Tooth disease; and Christopher Goetz of Rush University in Chicago for helping out on the historical Charcot. Tim White of the University of California at Berkeley shared his expertise on paleoarcheology, and Rosalind Ridley was generous with her firsthand knowledge of the history of prion diseases. She was present at the creation. I would also like to acknowledge a debt to her book, *Fatal Protein,* co-written with her husband, Harry Baker (New York: Oxford, 1998), from which I got my first education on the field.

Additional research help was kindly provided by a scrum of journalists and graduate students picked up in strange places along this book's journey, among them, in the rough order in which I met them: Daisy Prince, Christian Hunter, Maya Ponte, Anya Kamenetz, Marcelo Ortigao, Laila Weir, Marcel Schmidt, Kirsten Jackson, Alan Wirzbicki, and Amos Kenigsberg. Mario Sartor bicycled me, and Sabrina Marconi drove me, around the Veneto. The writer Philip Weiss, doing his own work in Papua New Guinea, kept one eye out on my behalf and on return read an early draft of this book, his suggestions helping to make it better.

Two research collection librarians came to my aid at key moments: at the Mandeville Special Collections Library at the University of San Diego, Kathy Creely dug through patrol reports, and at the Sutro library in San Francisco Martha Whittaker explored the mysterious contents of the Joseph Banks wool papers box. I also wish to thank Neil Chambers, her counterpart at the Natural History Museum in London. May the two of you meet one day! Oxonian Jennifer Quilter—a John Ashbery scholar, of all things—did a remarkable job of finding out about modern British cattle feeding practices. I also want to thank three Italian historians: Ernesto Gallo for his deep knowledge of the history of the town in which the Italian family lives; Andrea Peressini for his research on the Venetian doctor; and Achille Giachino for sharing his expert knowledge of eighteenth-century Venetian medicine. Finally, Nicoletta Pireddu of Georgetown University helped answer many questions of Italian culture and treacherous Italian grammar, as did my late beloved uncle, the playwright Jerry Max.

The list of those who were kind enough to cooperate with interviews is a long one and I have omitted some who did not want to be identified: among those connected to the kuru story, Michael Alpers, Paul Brown, Judith Farquhar, D. Carleton Gajdusek, William Hadlow, Igor Klatzo, Shirley Lindenbaum, and Gunther Stent; in Oceania, Hank Nelson of the Australian National University and patrol officers Jack Baker, Patrick Dwyer, and Jim Sinclair; among those involved in the mad cow story, David Bee, Gerald Bradley, John Collinge, Stephen Dealler, Alan Dickinson, Hugh Fraser, James Ironside, Howard Rees, Carol Richardson, Colin Whittaker, and Raymond Williams; on variant CJD in Britain, Donald Simms and Graham Steel of the CJD Alliance; for sharing variant CJD documents, Maureen Treadwell; among those who play a role in the CWD story and the threat of mad cow here, Peter Crino, Allen Mahan, Gene Schoonveld, Terry Singeltary (who has proven a loyal friend to this book over the years), and Janet Skarbek; for general help in the often obscure world of prion science, Byron Caughey of the NIH, Susan Lindquist of the Whitehead Institute at MIT, A. C. Palmer of Cambridge University, Bob Peterson of Case Western, and Charles Weissman of the Scripps Research Institute; on population genetics, David Goldstein of University College, London; at the University of San Francisco, Fred Cohen, Stephen D'Armond, the gracious Michael Geschwind, and Stanley Prusiner (fitfully); at Cold Spring Harbor Laboratory, James Watson via e-mail; on self-assembling systems, the always-generous Shuguang Zhang of MIT.

I would like to thank five writers who went before me for generously sharing knowledge and documents: Robert Draper, author of "The Genius Who Loved Boys" (*GQ,* November 1999); Maxime Schwartz, author of *How the Cows Turned Mad* (Berkeley, California: UC Berkeley Press, 2003); Gary Taubes, the author of a famous take-down of Stanley Prusiner, "The Name of the Game Is Fame but Is It Science?" (*Discover,* December 1986); Claudia Winkler, author of "Ignoble Nobelman" (*Weekly Standard,* October 7, 1996); and Roger J. Wood and

Vitezslaw Orel, authors of *Genetic Prehistory in Selective Breeding* (New York: Oxford University Press, 2001).

Many people lent me shelter and tea while I researched and wrote this moveable deadly feast of a book, among them Lisa Gabor, Carmen Greenebaum, Maurice and Jessica Hochschild, my brother and sister-in-law Adam and Diane Max, Barbara Thomas, and two bakeries: the Firehook Bakery and the wondrous St. Elmo's of Alexandria, Virginia.

To my agent, Elyse Cheney, her assistant, Stephanie Hanson, her colleague Peter McGuigan and their associates at the Abner Stein Agency in London, my heartfelt gratitude for their endless work in getting this book to readers. And to the editors who took this book from first idea to finished volume—Daniel Zalewski, Daniel Menaker, James Ryerson, and Lisa Chase—I would have considered myself lucky to have met one of you, let alone all four. Finally, I dedicate this book to the memory of Robert Jones, its acquiring editor, who showed the courage mixed with acceptance in the face of disease that this book is about.

NOTES

A NOTE ON SOURCES

I have tried to keep my notes short while providing a comprehensible if not comprehensive trail for the reader wishing to go deeper. Most of the quotations in
the book come from interviews I conducted; where not, I have cited the source
in the notes below. Also I have given a citation where I have either been particularly dependent on another's work or am quoting from that work. However, if a
written source is well known and easily available and searchable on the Web—
say, Bentham's *Fragment on Government* on page 21—I did not annotate.

Attributions and annotations for the Italian portions of this book presented
a different challenge. For one thing, I agreed to keep the last name of the family
with fatal familial insomnia private. In addition, little had been written on them
before I met them, so there are no published sources to cite. The facts relating to
their story are based on their memories, supplemented by letters, newspaper reports, civic documents, medical and other records they shared with me, and,
where possible, diaries, and interviews with other participants. The chapter on
the Venetian doctor, the first family member who may have had the disease, is by
definition speculative (though I have tried to present the historical and medical
background accurately). Confirmation that he was the first, the "Patient Zero,"
awaits research now underway by the family. The identity of Patient Zero has
changed before and may change again. The other chapters on the family rely on
documented sources. If a family member has a thought or emotion or says something in these pages, I know this either because they wrote it down or talked

about it with close relatives at the time. Their story is written to be literally true and as accurate as I could make it.

I of course take responsibility for any errors.

ABBREVIATIONS OF FREQUENTLY CITED BOOKS

PDHA: *Prion Diseases of Humans and Animals,* edited by Stanley Prusiner, John Collinge, et al. (Chichester, England: Ellis Horwood, 1992).

KURU: *Early Letters and Field Notes from the Collection of D. Carleton Gajdusek,* edited by Gajdusek and Judith Farquhar (New York: Raven Press, 1981).

JFN: Carleton Gajdusek, *1955–1957 Journal and Field Notes: Australia, Territory of Papua and Trust Territory of New Guinea* (Bethesda, Maryland: National Institutes of Health, 1996).

KEP: Carleton Gajdusek, *Kuru Epidemiological Patrol from the New Guinea Highlands to Papua, August 21, 1957–November 10, 1957* (Bethesda, Maryland: National Institutes of Health, 1963).

INTRODUCTION

xiii *"almost immortal":* The researcher was Paul Brown of the NIH, interviewed in *The Brain Eater,* broadcast on PBS on February 10, 1998.

xiv *"effective therapy":* "Neurologist Says Nobel Prize Supports Work," Reuters Online Service, October 6, 1997.

xiv *in five years:* Judy Siegel-Itzkovich, "A 'Crazy Idea' That Happened to Be True," *Jerusalem Post,* May 24, 1998.

xviii *"If sleep does not serve":* quoted in *Fatal Familial Insomnia: Inherited Prion Diseases, Sleep, and the Thalamus,* Christian Guilleminault et al., eds. (New York: Raven Press, 1995), p. xiii.

xviii *"Then I went to sleep":* Randy Gardner, ". . . To Stay Awake for Eleven Days," *Esquire,* Vol. 142.2 (August 2004), p. 87.

xix *Allan Rechtschaffen came close:* The experiment was conducted in his University of Chicago lab in the 1960s. A. Rechtschaffen, et al. "Physiological Correlates of Prolonged Sleep Deprivation in Rats," *Science,* 221 (July 8, 1983), pp. 182–84.

xix *recent scientific studies:* Laske, et al., "The Effect of Stress on the Onset and Progression of Creutzfeldt-Jakob Disease: Results of a German Pilot Case-Control Study," *European Journal of Epidemiology,* Vol. 15, No. 7 (August 1999), pp. 631–35.

xxv *dismissive words:* Charles Tanford and Jacqueline Reynolds, *Nature's Robots: A History of Proteins* (New York: Oxford University Press, 2001).

xxvi *A recent proteomics conference:* quoted in Carol Ezzell, "Proteins Rule," *Scientific American,* Vol. 286, Issue 4 (April 2002), p. 42.

xxvi *"My husband seen":* posted on www.CJDVoice.org, October 27, 1998.

xxviii *"The coroner here":* posted on www.CJDVoice.org, November 11, 1998.

xxix *"there was only some way":* posted on www.CJDVoice.org, January 2, 2006.

CHAPTER 1: **THE DOCTORS' DILEMMA**

4 *Venice's fall:* For the discussion of eighteenth-century Venice, I am indebted to Pompeo Molmenti's *La storia di Venezia nella vita privata dalle origini alla caduta della repubblica* (Bergamo, Italy: Istituto italiano d'arti grafiche, 1905–1908), especially Volume III, on the decadent end of the Serenissima, where one may find, among other facts, that there were 852 barbers and wigmakers in Venice at the fall of the Republic. A shortened version of this great work was published in America in 1906, translated by Horatio F. Brown. I also owe a debt to Paolo Scandaletti's *La Venezia è caduta* (Venice: Neri Pozza, 1997) and *Venezia e l'esperienza 'democratica' del 1797* (Venice: Ateneo Veneto, 1997), edited by Stefano Pillinini.

4 *Its ruling class:* The Venetians were always eager for money, so they occasionally opened the book of nobility to admit families that made significant financial contributions—a minimum of 100,5 ducats—to the state. But they never forgot the difference between the new nobles and their own more august selves.

5 *The scientific method:* Among recent achievements at Padua were the first accurate drawings of the body (Vesalius), the discovery that blood circulates (Harvey), the first studies of pathological anatomy (Morgagni), not to mention definitive proof against Aristotle's idea of spontaneous generation. In 1668, Francesco Redi showed that the reason one found maggots on rotten meat was not that they had spontaneously generated there but

that flies had laid their eggs on it. Pasteur was doing little more than confirming Redi's theory with his goosenecked flasks two hundred years later.

5   *"Science,"he had written:* Galileo, *Il Saggiatore* (1623), my translation.

6   *a "high funnel":* Goethe, *Travels in Italy,* September 27, 1786, W. H. Auden and Elizabeth Mayer, translators (London: Wm. Collins, 1962), p. 71.

9   *gyrate wildly:* Fever in FFI victims is caused by the damage prions do to the thalamus, which regulates body temperature, rather than by the body's attempt to fight off infection. In prion diseases where the thalamus is not damaged, there is typically no fever.

9   *They had all suffered humiliations:* The story appears in Chapter 7 of Casanova's far-from-reliable memoirs.

10   *"Who is it that says":* Arthur Young, *Travels in Italy and France* (New York: Everyman, nd), p. 63.

10   *The Venetians had begun manufacturing:* A typical 1787 advertisement from a Venetian pharmacy for *Theriaca ex Galeno* lists thirty ingredients, including *Iunci Arabii* and *Dictamni Cretici* (roughly, gum Arabic and Cretan dittany bark). Found in Nelli-Elena Vanzan Marchini, ed., *Dalla scienza medica alla pratica dei corpi* (Venice: Neri Pozza, 1993), p. 178.

11   *"the base and foundation . . .":* The Aldrovandi quote can be found in Giuseppe Olmi's "Farmacopia Antica e Medicina Moderna," from *Physis* (1977), my translation, p. 203.

12   *"A Venetian law lasts but a week":* The speaker was Girolamo Priuli, in the early sixteenth century. The story of the Venetian response to occupation can be found in both *Venezia e l'esperienza* and *Venezia Suddita,* ed. Michele Gottardi (Venice: Ateneo Veneto, 1999).

14   *one quarter of the residents:* The figure is from the 1849 Austrian military inquiry into malaria in the Veneto. (Cited in *"Mal aere" e "malaria,"* A. Canalis and P. Sepulcri, eds. [Rome: Tipografia Regionale, 1961], p. 1042.) Wrote one concerned member of an investigating group, Count M. A. Sanfermo, two years before, "Whoever cares to look at the large zone that surrounds the Adriatic will see nothing but vast almost deserted tracts of land, where a few unhappy souls eek out an existence between squalor and misery. Three hundred thousand *campi* offer the unwelcome aspect of unhealthy and unhappy marshland." *"Mal aere,"* my transaltion, p. 1037.

14   *The local witch:* I am indebted to Roberta Purisiol's thesis *La medicina nell'entroterra veneziano* for information on attitudes toward sickness and

alternative healing in the Veneto in the eighteenth century (published in the series *Quaderni di Studi e Notizie* [Mestre, Italy: Centro Studi Storici di Mestre, nd]).

16 *encephalitis lethargica:* An excellent general introduction to the epidemic can be found in the opening chapter of Oliver Sacks's *Awakenings* (New York: Summit Press, 1987).

17 *Because large families:* There is no agreement on why this may be. Indeed, some researchers think the imbalance is an artifact of the reality that large families with mutations tend to receive more research attention, because they make better subjects for genetic studies. It is at least true in the FFI family that the poorest branches are by far the hardest hit by the disease.

CHAPTER 2: **MERINO MANIA**

19 *"Machines for converting":* quoted in John Sinclair, *The Code of Agriculture* (London, Sherwood Gilbert and Piper, 1832; first edition, 1817), p. 83. (Cited in *Genetic Prehistory in Selective Breeding* by Roger J. Wood and Vitezslaw Orel [New York: Oxford University Press, 2001], p. 78.)

21 *The spirit of the age:* For information on Bakewell's life, I relied on H. C. Pawson's *Robert Bakewell* (London: Crosby Lockwood, 1957) as well as Wood and Orel's *Genetic Prehistory in Selective Breeding.*

23 *"setting themselves in opposition":* Richard Parkinson, *Treatise on the Breeding and Management of Livestock* (London: Cadell & Davies, 1810), p. 267.

23 *"substitute[d] profitable flesh":* Anonymous [John Lawrence], "Robert Bakewell" in *The Annual Necrology for 1797–1798 Including Various Articles of Neglected Biography* (London: R. Phillips, 1800), p. 205. (Cited in Wood and Orel, *Genetic Prehistory,* p. 75.)

23 *Drawn by Young's publicity:* Bakewell's fame crossed even the Atlantic; in 1787, George Washington ordered farm implements from him, hoping for a touch of his magic.

24 *Even so, the gentry:* My discussion of Joseph Banks—as well as many of the quotations in these pages—are drawn in part from H. B. Carter's *His Majesty's Spanish Flock* (Sydney: Angus & Robertson, 1964) and from the collection of correspondence edited by Carter, *The Sheep and Wool Correspondence of Sir Joseph Banks, 1781–1820* (New South Wales: Library Council, 1979).

24 *"a Newcastle coal-heaver":* Epicurus (pseud.), "Letter from a Farmer," *Farmer's Magazine,* 4 (October 1802), pp. 35-37. (Cited in Wood and Orel, *Genetic Prehistory,* p. 109.)

25 *Boys inherited the job of shepherd:* William Youatt, an expert on husbandry, wrote of the Mesta shepherds, "They are a singular race of men, enthusiastically attracted to their profession, rarely quitting it, even for a more lucrative one, and rarely marrying." *Sheep: Their Breeds, Management, and Diseases* (London: Baldwin and Cradock, 1837), p. 153.

25– *"a peculiar coarse"; "a singular looseness of the skin":* Youatt, *Sheep: Their*
26 *Breeds,* both p. 148.

27 *merinos "in almost every district of Great Britain":* quoted by C. P. Lasteyrie in *Histoire de l'introduction des moutons à laine fine d'Espagne dan les divers états de l'Europe, et au cap du Bonne-Espérance* (Paris, 1802), translated by Benjamin Thompson as "An Account of the Introduction of Merino Sheep into the Different States of Europe, and at the Cape of Good Hope (London: J. Harding, 1810), p. 143.

28 *"No person who has taste":* in Comber's *Real Improvements in Agriculture (On the Principles of A. Young, Esq.) Recommended to Accompany Improvements of Rents.* Few details of Comber's life have come down to us; however, being a narcissist, he could not avoid autobiography in his writings.

29 *"a fixed and convulsed position":* Hogg is better known today for his 1824 Gothic novel *The Private Memoirs and Confessions of a Justified Sinner.*

29 *He got a London printer:* W. Nicoll of St. Paul's Church Yard, London.

30 *disease was local:* I am indebted for some of these terms to J. P. McGowan's *Investigation into the Disease of Sheep called "Scrapie"* (Edinburgh: Blackwood & Sons: 1914), p. 10. McGowan's work is the beginning text for modern historical scrapie studies.

31 *"bad taste & unnatural pride":* quotation is from a letter from John White Parsons to Banks (1800), quoted in Carter, *His Majesty's Spanish Flock,* p. 273.

31 *references to "goggles" and the "mad staggers":* Some mentions can be found in H. B. Carter's *His Majesty's Spanish Flock.* Others are in the uncatalogued Joseph Banks papers at the Sutro library, located at the University of California–San Francisco.

32 *"kill it immediately":* The writer was Johann Georg Stumpf, "An Essay on the Practical History of Sheep in Spain," in *Transactions of the Royal*

Dublin Society (Dublin: Graisberry & Campbell, 1800), translated from a German edition of 1785 by the Rev. Dr. Lanigan, p. 98.

32 *In what is probably:* The writer, a clergyman, invokes the disease in advising Christians to mix with heathen: "In a word as it is wholesome for a flock of sheep for some goats to feed amongst them, their bad sent being good Phisique for the sheep to keep them from the Shakings; so much profit rebounds to the Godly by the necessary mixture of the wicked amongst them, making the pious to stick the faster to God and Goodness." Thomas Fuller, *The Holy State and the Profane State* (Cambridge: Printed by R. Daniel for J. Williams, 1642), p. 401.

32 *Edward Lisle:* His comments on scrapie come in his "Observations in Husbandry," published after his death by his son (London: J. Hughs, 2nd edition, 1757).

33 *"Disease is that deviation from health":* Vial de Sainbel, *Elements of the Veterinary Art* (London: J. Wright, 1797), p. 3. For an idea of how primitive human medicine remained, consider this treatment for dog bite offered by the leading Scottish medical journal in 1825: "Treatment of person bitten by mad dogs: Deep scarifications of the wound, besmearing it with the pulvis lyttae, application of a blister in the neighbourhood of the part, keeping up of suppuration, both in the blistered and the wounded part, during six weeks, and the rubbing in of mercurial ointment till symptoms of approaching salivation come on. . . . If the clothes are also bitten through, they are always burnt." The journal, the *Medical and Surgical Journal,* comments that of 233 rabies sufferers thus treated, only 4 died.

34 *"regained his gaiety and his appetite":* Hénon, "Sur la cause de la maladie du mouton, désignée sous le nom de vertige ou tournoiement," *Mémoirs et Observations sur La Chirurgie* (c. 1800), my translation, p. 404.

35 *The mite took twelve days:* A.K.S. Von Richthofen, "On Distinguishing the Trotting Disease from the Rot in Sheep" (Korn, 1827).

36 *"violent ardor, incompletely satisfied":* J. Girard, "Notice sur quelques maladie peu connue des bêtes à laine," *Recueil de médicine vétérinaire,* Vol. 7 (1830), p. 32. Other writers associate scrapie with sheep prone to "onanism." (Cited in McGowan, *Investigation,* p. 18.)

36 *"tumours of a size varying":* A. Bénion, "Traité complet de l'elevage et des maladies du mouton" (Paris, 1874), p. 444. (Translated and cited by McGowan, *Investigation,* pp. 28–29.)

36 *"our luckless farmers"*: letter from M. Roche-Lubin to the editor of the *Recueil de médicine vétérinaire,* June 2, 1835, quoted in Martin Villemin, *Les Vétérinaires français au XIXe siècle* (Maisons-Alfort, France: Editions du Point Veterinaire, 1982), my translation, p. 245.

36 "ni ulcères, ni vésicules": Just Cauvet, "Sur la tremblante," *Journal des vétérinaires du Midi* (1854), p. 442.

36 *"true causes"*: M. Roche-Lubin, "Mémoire pratique sur la maladie des bêtes à laine connue sous les noms de prurigo lombaire, convulsive, trembleuse, tremblante, etc.," *Recueil de medicine vétérinaire* (1848), my translation, pp. 698–714.

37 "Nous avons énoncé": J. Girard, "Notice sur quelques maladies," p. 70.

37 *"the* rubbers": Arthur Young, *General View of the Agriculture of Lincolnshire* (London, second edition, 1813), p. 372.

37 *"an obscure disease of sheep"*: S. Stockman, *Journal of Comparative Pathology and Therapeutics* (1913), pp. 317–27.

CHAPTER 3: **PIETRO**

40 *A joke:* The Austrian statesmen Metternich memorably described Italy as more a geographical expression than a country.

48 *"Anatomy"*: Emil Kraepelin made the comment to the physician Oskar Vogt in 1894. Found in *The Founders of Neurology,* Webb Haymaker, ed. (Springfield, Ill.: C.C. Thomas, 1953), p. 165.

49 *On autopsy, the victims:* In the 1980s, a group led by Carleton Gajdusek reexamined the slides and concluded that none of Creutzfeldt's patients had CJD and only some of Jakob's did. See "The Spectrum of Creutzfeldt-Jakob Disease and the Virus-Induced Subacute Spongiform Encephalopathies," *Recent Advances in Neuropathology 2* (Edinburgh: Churchill Livingstone, 1982), p. 139.

CHAPTER 4: **STRONG MAGIC**

53 *"Young man, be careful!"*: quoted in Vincent Zigas, *Laughing Death* (Totowa, New Jersey: Humana Press, 1990), p. 22.

55 *One day R. I. Skinner:* The story is told in Shirley Lindenbaum's *Kuru Sorcery* (Mountain View, California: Mayfield, 1979), p. 80. Retired patrol

officers dispute whether Skinner patrolled with a machine gun or just a pistol.

57 *"The natives received us":* A. T. Carey, patrol report #1, Goroka and Kratke subdistricts, 1951-52, p. 2. The patrol reports cited in these notes are all on microfilm at the Mandeville Special Collections Library, University of California, San Diego, in La Jolla. All the reports are from the Eastern Highlands patrol region.

58 *the suspicion:* "It was surprising, that in this area which has no ready access to medical attention, should be so free from serious cases of disease," patrol officer W. J. Kelly wrote in early October 1953. Patrol report #6, Kainantu subdistrict, 1953-54, p. 5.

58 *"a hole in the ground":* John McArthur, patrol report #4, Kainantu subdistrict, 1954-55, p. 13. The latrine depth was a long-standing problem. "To be effective the hole must be of considerable depth," Tiny Carey lectured the Fore in 1949. A. T. Carey, report #3, Goroka subdistrict, 1949-50, p. 5.

58 *"It appears":* A. T. Carey, patrol report # 4, Goroka subdistrict, 1950-51 (August 15-21, 1950), p. 5.

59 *"Nearing one of the dwellings":* J. R. McArthur, patrol report #10, Goroka subdistrict, 1953-54, p. 3.

59 *"bottomless":* John Colman, patrol report #14, Kainantu subdistrict, 1954-55, p. 8.

60 *Then he threatened with arrest:* J. R. McArthur, patrol report #4, Kainantu subdistrict, 1954-55, p. 10.

60 *put a sorcery bundle in his mouth:* John Colman, patrol report #14, Kainantu subdistrict, 1954-55, p. 6.

60 *"romanticism of the Central European": JFN,* June 30, 1956.

60 *highly embellished memoirs:* Zigas's two memoirs are *Auscultation of Two Worlds* (1978), which he self-published, and *Laughing Death.* The story of Apekono and McArthur can be found in the latter, pp. 122-33.

62 *"an attitude of intense dislike":* J. A. Wiltshire, patrol report #8, Okapa subdistrict, Eastern Highlands, 1959-60, p. 7.

62 *confiscated the charm:* J. C. Baker, patrol report #7, Kainantu subdistrict, 1956-57, p. 4.

62 *six hundred deaths:* Ibid.

64 *"Try to find one":* The societal strain kuru put the Fore under is recounted in Lindenbaum, *Kuru Sorcery.*

64 *"to look after it":* Ibid, p. 102.

CHAPTER 5: **DOCTA AMERICA**

67 *On the morning:* Information on Carleton Gajdusek comes in part from his voluminous diaries, which he published through his office at the NIH, as well as from biographical material and interviews with Gajdusek and his former colleagues.

68 *"You're a screwball":* quoted by Gajdusek in Carleton Gajdusek, *Expedition to the Flooded Uruma Settlement of Okinawan Colonists on the Rio Guapai, Amazonas of Bolivia to Search for the Etiology of Fatal Jungle Fever. . . .* March 10, 1955–March 18, 1955, in the collection of the American Philosophical Library, Philadelphia, Pennsylvania.

68 *"In the slow routine": JFN,* December 15, 1955.

69 *at "two guineas a day": JFN,* March 8, 1957.

69 *"The whole setting": JFN,* March 9, 1957.

69 *"I pray": JFN,* November 14, 1955.

70 *"Few master this surf!": JFN,* April [nd], 1956.

70 *His journals:* Gajdusek restricts a few, which he says are more explicit, but Judith Farquhar, who edited many of the journals and has seen the restricted material, says it is no more suggestive than that which was published, lending credence to the idea that Gajdusek's sex life was in large part in his imagination. As Farquhar puts it, Gajdusek had "a very interesting kind of generalized erotic stance on the world. An endless passionate interest in people, things, ideas, books, scientific facts, everything. He probably didn't narrow his desire very often to individual people, particular 'sex acts.' The French philosopher Gilles Deleuze said 'we always make love with worlds' " (e-mail to me).

70 *"Little to write of": JFN,* February 20, 1956.

70 *"I frankly am shopping":* D. Carleton Gajdusek, ed., *Correspondence on the Discovery and Original Investigations on Kuru* (Bethesda, Maryland: NIH, 1975). Gajdusek to Smadel, September 28, 1956.

71 *"leave it out": Correspondence,* Smadel to Gajdusek, March 6, 1956.

71 *Besides his wanderlust:* Gajdusek has gone on to write another sixty volumes, in addition to almost a thousand scientific papers.

71 *Sir Mac was tired:* Burnet, himself an interesting figure who was instrumental in placing Australian on par with European medicine, wrote an autobiography, *Changing Patterns* (London: William Heinemann, 1968),

notable for mentioning his tormentor Gajdusek only once in almost three hundred pages.

72 *"Bitter? No?": JFN,* March 8, 1957.

72 *"possible dangers from hostile native reaction": Kuru,* Burnet to John T. Gunther, February 12, 1957.

72 *waiting for an answer: Kuru,* Gunther to Burnet, February 15, 1957.

72 *He could inspire Zigas:* Zigas wound up working for Gajdusek at the National Institutes of Health, in Bethesda, Maryland, and died of a mysterious brain ailment in 1983.

73 *"another American invasion":* Notes taken by Sir Mac of a conversation with Scragg, cited in *Kuru,* March 29, 1957.

73 *"Women and children": JFN,* March 6, 1957.

73 *"[Zigas] tells me that all": Kuru,* Gajdusek to Burnet, Ian Wood and Anderson, March 13, 1957.

73 *"informed of our every move": Kuru,* Gajdusek to Burnet, April 20, 1957.

73 *"Intensive investigation uninterruptible": Kuru,* Gajdusek to Scragg, nd, p. 28.

74 *"We are lab minded": Kuru,* Gajdusek to Scragg, April 6, 1957.

74 *"emotional instability": Kuru,* Gajdusek to Smadel, July 25, 1957.

74 *"Could any more astounding": Kuru,* Gajdusek to Smadel, May 28, 1957.

75 *"post-encephalitis": Kuru,* Gajdusek to Scragg, March 20, 1957.

76 *"one of the most mystifying": Kuru,* Gajdusek to Smadel, August 6, 1957.

76 *"great pig-tusks": Kuru,* Gajdusek to Smadel, August 25, 1957.

77 *"very spectacular neuronophagia": Kuru,* Klatzo to Smadel, August 15, 1957.

77 *"described by Jakob and Creutzfeldt": Kuru,* Klatzo to Gajdusek, September 15, 1957.

77 *"Two cases": Kuru,* Gajdusek to Smadel, September 18, 1957.

77 *"The natives evinced": Kuru,* Gajdusek to J. Baker, Zigas, and [field dietician Lucy] Hamilton, September 8, 1957.

77 *"a first-rate scientist": Kuru,* Burnet to Gunther, April (nd), 1957, p. 41.

77 *"with experts in anthropology": Kuru,* Imus to Smadel, August 8, 1957.

78 *"In the eastern": Time* (November 11, 1957), p. 55.

78 *"ready to bleed Kuks galore": Kuru,* Gajdusek to Roy T. Simmons, November 12, 1957.

78 *"Joseph Conrad, American verse": Kuru,* September 11, 1957.

78 *"insistent and repeated offers of fellatio"*: *KEP,* October 7, 1957. Gajdusek published these passages as I have recorded them in his first version of the kuru story in 1963 but edited part of them out of subsequent, more widely available versions.

79 *"wonderful Kukukukus"*: *Kuru,* Gajdusek to Smadel, November 4, 1957.

79 *"some good!!"*: Gajdusek was writing from Hollandia, on the Western, or Dutch, side of New Guinea. *Kuru,* January 28, 1958.

79 *Evolutionary theory:* The classic instance of a genetic disease that compensates for its potential lethality with a benefit is sickle-cell anemia, which also confers protection against malaria.

79 *"my overseas guest, the two belles"*: *Auscultation,* p. 164.

81 *"cheerfully admit[ing]"*: R. I. Skinner, patrol report #5, Kainantu subdistrict, 1947–48.

81 *As one Fore described the process:* recounted in Ronald Berndt, *Excess and Restraint* (Chicago: University of Chicago Press, 1962), p. 271. [Berndt was one of the first anthropologists in the region.]

82 *"That humans could be food"*: Lindenbaum, *Kuru Sorcery,* ch. 4, to which I am indebted for the understanding of the relationship between the Fore and food and the details of their endocannibalistic feasts. Another source is Berndt's *Excess.*

82 *"I eat you"*: recounted in Berndt, *Excess,* p. viii. An almost identical moment appears in W. J. Kelly's patrol report #8, Kainantu subdistrict, 1951–52, Appendix B, where he describes the Fore assessing the "possible protein value of the patrol."

83 *"The South Fore adults and children"*: *JFN,* March 9, 1957. (This comment by Gajdusek first appears in *JFN* in 1996. Gajdusek had omitted it from previous journal publications covering the period.)

83 *A week later: Kuru,* Gajdusek to Smadel, March 15, 1957.

CHAPTER 6: **MONKEY BUSINESS**

86 *a flock of sheep in Michigan:* The diagnosing veterinarian wrote with surprise, "When the hand was placed upon the lumbar region and the area palpated with the fingers, the 'scratch reflex' was very noticeable, being manifested by nibbling movements of the lips." F. Thorp, et al., "Scrapie in Sheep," *Michigan State College Veterinarian* (Fall 1952), pp. 86–87.

86 *"overall resemblance":* Hadlow, "The Scrapie-Kuru Connection: Recollection of How It Came About," *PDHA,* p. 43.

86 *"the one person":* Ibid.

86 *In the 1930s:* The two French veterinarians were L. Cuille and P. L. Chelle, whose works make nice bookends. "La maladie dite tremblante du mouton est-elle inoculable?" and "La tremblant du mouton est bien inoculable." Both in *Comptes rendus de l'Académie des Sciences* (Paris: published in 1936 and 1939, respectively).

88 *"exalted handler of apes":* Hadlow, "Scrapie-Kuru Connection," *PDHA,* p. 44.

89 *Gibbs complemented:* CJD family members thought so highly of Gibbs that they created a memorial for him on www.CJDVoice.org after his death in 2001.

89 *"before five years":* Gajdusek and C. J. Gibbs, "Attempts to Demonstrate a Transmissible Agent in Kuru, Amyotrophic Lateral Sclerosis, and Other Sub-acute and Chronic System Degenerations of Man," *Nature,* Vol. 204 (October 1964), pp. 257–59.

90 *"a plethora":* C. J. Gibbs, "Spongiform Encephalopathies—Slow, Latent, and Temperate Virus Infections—in Retrospect," *PDHA,* p. 59. Jared Diamond, the well-known science writer, had a less cheerful view of the facilities. In his book *The Third Chimpanzee,* he recalls seeing a chimpanzee at Patuxent "injected with a slow-acting lethal virus . . . being kept alone for the several years until it died, in a small indoor cage devoid of play objects." Jared Diamond, *The Third Chimpanzee* (New York: HarperCollins, 1992), p. 31.

90 *"in the terminal phase":* Michael Alpers, "Kuru: Implications of Its Transmissibility for the Interpretation of its Changing Epidemiological Pattern" in *The Central Nervous System,* O. T. Baile and D. E. Smith, eds. (Baltimore: Williams and Wilkins, 1968), p. 241.

91 *C. J. Gibbs says:* in "Spongiform Encephalopathies," *PDHA,* p. 60. Gajdusek made his claim in an interview with me.

92 *One British committee recommended:* Agricultural Research Council, "Report of the Advisory Committee on Scrapie" (October 12, 1976), p. 4.

92 *The South African–born radiologist:* Alper also took a gun off a mugger when she was past eighty. (Judy Goodkin, "Public Lives: Up and Atom," *The Guardian* [April 29, 1992].) Her intimidating presence at talks and lectures is still remembered by British scientists.

93 *"a well-known virus":* D. Carleton Gajdusek, "Unconventional Viruses and the Origin and Disappearance of Kuru" in *Science,* Vol. 197 (4307) (September 2, 1977), pp. 943-60.

94 *"dismissed as buffoonery":* I. H. Pattison, "A Sideways Look at the Scrapie Saga: 1961-1981," *PDHA,* p. 21.

94 *he posited three ways:* J. S. Griffith, "Self-Replication and Scrapie," *Nature,* Vol. 215 (105) (1967), pp. 1043-44.

96 *Gajdusek had a theory:* Gajdusek, "Unconventional Viruses," p. 958.

CHAPTER 8: **A WONDERFUL PROBLEM FOR A CHEMIST**

116 *As he pointed out:* Gary Taubes, "The Name of the Game Is Fame but Is It Science?" *Discover,* Vol. 7 (December 1986) pp. 28-52.

116 *In 1984, he bragged:* Stanley Prusiner, "Prions," *Scientific American,* Vol. 251 (October 1984), pp. 50-59.

118 *Prusiner chronicled his progress:* To take three papers published in short order; "Sedimentation Properties of the Scrapie Agent," in the *Proceedings of the National Academy of Sciences* (Vol. 74, October 1977, pp. 4661-65); "Suppression of Polyclonal B Cell Activation in Scrapie-infected C3H/HeJ Mice," in the *Journal of Immunology* (Vol. 120 [6] June 1978, pp. 1986-90); and "Experimental Scrapie in Mice: Ultrastructural Observations" in *Annals of Neurology* (v. 4 [3], September 1978, pp. 205-11). One cannot imagine Gajdusek putting his name to such work, even as senior author.

119 *This system works only:* Taubes, "The Name of the Game."

120 *pressing Congress:* statement to the Food Safety Caucus, House of Representatives, January 27, 2004.

120 *eating a T-bone steak:* University of San Francisco Office of Press Information.

120 *The divorce papers:* filed in California Superior Court (Prusiner v. Prusiner, case #: FL 036246).

121 Nature *called it:* "Nobel Panel Rewards Prion Theory After Years of Heated Debate." *Nature,* Vol. 389 (6551) (October 9, 1997), p. 529.

122 *The word did have:* Frederic Wood Jones, "Lady Percy Island," *Discovery* (London), Vol. 18 (209) (May 1937), p. 141.

123 *"Tiny Life Form Found":* David Perlman, *San Francisco Chronicle,* February 19, 1982.

126 *"persuasive experiment"*: Stanley Prusiner, "The Prion Diseases," *Scientific American,* Vol. 272 (January 1995), pp. 48–57.

127 *sporadic, infectious, and genetic:* The disease that comes closest is cancer, but no single cancer can occur in all three ways, as, say, Creutzfeldt-Jakob disease can.

127 *convert the normal one:* Byron Caughey, "Cell-Free Formation of Protease-Resistant Prion Protein," *Nature,* Vol. 370 (6489) (August 11, 1994), pp. 471–74.

129 *James Watson does not agree:* e-mail to me, June 30, 2005.

129 *"We have compelling evidence":* Sandra Blakeslee, "Study Lends Support to Mad Cow Theory," *The New York Times,* July 30, 2004.

CHAPTER 9: **CONVERGENCE**

135 *In 1953:* One reason it took researchers so long to discover REM is that it does not take place at the beginning of the sleep cycle, so if the researcher himself nods off, he misses the phenomenon.

141 *maximum reading on his thermometer:* Remarkably, considering the events that preceded it, the hospital recorded the cause of death as meningitis.

146 *Prusiner had successfully shown:* The key paper is "Evidence for the Conformation of the Pathologic Isoform of the Prion Protein Enciphering and Propagating Prion Diversity." *Science,* Vol. 274 (5295) (December 20, 1996), pp. 2079–82.

146 *"There are still people":* quoted in Lawrence K. Altman, "U.S. Scientist Wins Nobel for Controversial Work," *The New York Times,* October 7, 1997.

147 *"an eye opening acquaintance":* D. Carleton Gajdusek, *The Decline and Fall of Prospect Hill: The End of a Decade of Manorial Living* (Bethesda, Maryland: NIH, 1991), p. 61.

147 *"This case":* Robert Draper, "The Genius Who Loved Boys," *GQ,* Vol. 69 (11) (November 1999), pp. 313–30.

147 *"Gajdusek just started rambling":* unpublished interview with Montgomery County investigator, April 14, 1999. Courtesy of Robert Draper.

147 *"I don't care about":* Gajdusek investigation tapes, March 15, 1996. Courtesy of Robert Draper.

148 *fellate the boy:* The interview is recounted in an investigative report signed by a criminal investigator of the Frederick County, Maryland, felony division. Courtesy of Robert Draper.

148 *"didn't want to give up the gravy train":* unpublished interview, April 14, 1999. Courtesy of Robert Draper.

149 *"I never heard a word of original thought," Jail Journal,* 2nd ed. (Gif-sur-Yvonne, France: Institut Alfred Fessard, 2002) (October 30, 1997).

CHAPTER 10: **APOCALYPSE COW**

The story of the mad cow epidemic can be found in extraordinary detail in the record of the British government's investigation, called the BSE Inquiry (www.BSEinquiry.gov.uk), which includes much of the correspondence and notes of the participants. When I draw on these documents, I do not include an endnote. All quotations come either from my interviews with the participants or from their testimony to the BSE Inquiry.

155 *640 billion doses of BSE:* My estimate is a version of one made by Philip Yam, *The Pathological Protein* (New York: Springer-Verlag, 2003), p. 139, and is arrived at by multiplying the maximum estimated number of infected cows that went into the British food chain (1.6 million) by the maximum estimated number of people exposed to each cow consumed (400,000). The 400,000-person estimate comes from the European Union's scientific steering committee in 1999 and can be found at http://europa.eu.int/comm/food/fs/sc/ssc/out67_en.pdf.

157 "tête haute" *and* "regarde fixe": Roche-Lubin, "Mémoire," in *Recueil.*

160 *very excited:* Howard Rees, the chief veterinary officer, had a different response, as became clear during the BSE Inquiry. Asked by counsel for the Inquiry: "The scientists were enthusiastic, were they?" he replied, with a bureaucrat's condescension, "Of course they always are." Later a colleague reported seeing him leave the meeting at which he was given the news that scrapie had jumped to a cow "with steam pouring out of his ears." Accessed at http://www.bseinquiry.gov.uk/files/ws/s092t.pdf.

164 *"nutty"* . . . *"silly"* . . . *"bloody mad":* The first hint of what was to become a familiar nickname for the disease came in a report filed in January 1985 by the veterinary investigative officer who visited a suspect farm where workers had been trying to load a difficult animal on a truck to send it to be tested. "Cow went mad & aggressive," the official noted. The official questionnaire John Wilesmith prepared in 1987 for farmers who had had a BSE case in their flock used the term "maniacal." The *New Scientist,* a month later, was calling the cows "nutty" (Vol. 116 [1585], November 5,

1987). *The Star* a week after that asked, "Why [Are] the Cows So Silly?" in a headline. A reporter for *Farming News* interviewed an unnamed West Country farmer, who said that a cow in his herd had gone "bloody mad." The first national press printed mention appears to have been in a *Sunday Telegraph* story on November 6, 1988, titled "Virus Kills Prize Bull."

CHAPTER 11: OINKIES

170 *greatly and wondrously improved:* The *British Friesian Journal* notes with Bakewell-like pleasure: "Udders were improved in shape, durability and efficiency by leveling the hind-quarters and increasing their flatness, length and width. . . . Stamina or constitution was improved by breeding shorter legs under deeper bodies; by shortening the exceedingly long neck; by widening the nostrils and strengthening the jaws; by strengthening the topline so that the strongloin could support the well-sprung ribs which have to hold up the great barrel necessary to the capacious food storage associated with the exceptional milk-producer" (Vol. 28, June 1946, p. 125).

170 *"prepared to feed for the extra yield":* Dairy Farmer, July 1963.

170 *The man who first:* Readers interested in Liebig should turn to William H. Brock's *Justus von Liebig: The Chemical Gatekeeper* (New York: Cambridge University Press, 1997). Among his projects was a failed attempt in the 1860s to persuade the city of London to use its sewage to fertilize the surrounding crop lands.

171 *faint-feeling women:* Liebig's beef extract cube is still popular in England as Oxo and Bovril, and, on the Continent, as Liebig's.

171 *"refuse meat fibre":* Augustus Voelcker, "Annual Report of the Consulting Chemist for 1875," in *The Journal of the Royal Agricultural Society* (London: John Murray, 1876), pp. 293–94.

171 *Eventually, two kinds:* according to a German handbook by Martin Klimmer of Dresden, *Scientific Feeding of the Domestic Animals* (Chicago: A. Eger, 1923), translated by Paul Fischer.

171 *1909 scientific manual:* Oskar Kellner, *The Scientific Feeding of Animals* (New York: McMillan Company, 1909).

172 *"Are you mixing with the best?":* advertisement for Seemeel's H.B.F. Dairy Concentrate, cover of *Dairy Farmer,* October 1985.

176   *The winner was "Oinkies":* Meat and Livestock Commission press release, August 1, 1990.

179   *"DO NOT get mad cow":* Jojo Moyes, "Majors Assured Victim's Mother Meat Was Safe," *The Independent,* March 21, 1996.

179   *an inescapable conclusion:* Alan Watkins, "Why Is My Girl Dying?," *Today,* January 25, 1994.

179   *"I want my life back":* Anton Antonowicz, "Tragic Diary Note of Girl Doomed by Mad Cow Beefburger," *Daily Mirror,* January 26, 1997.

179   *dropped from sight:* Rimmer died in 1997. It was never proven that she had variant CJD. James Ironside, who had helped identify the first cases of variant CJD in the mid-1990s, called Rimmer's "one of the most unusual and difficult cases I have ever come across." Interview with the BBC, April 27, 2001.

180   *expressed his "astonishment":* John Major's comment was made to the president of the European Commission, Jacques Santer, reported in Patrick Wintour, et al., "Ministers Decry Beef Outcry," *The Guardian,* March 26, 1996.

180   *"Apocalypse Cow!":* Dairy Farmer, May 1996.

180   *"The housewife":* director of Anglo Beef Processors quoted in a 1996 report to the House of Commons entitled "Bovine Spongiform Encephalopathy and Creutzfeldt-Jakob Disease: Recent Developments."

181   *"rule out 500,000 cases":* John Pattison, quoted in "Epidemic," *Daily Mirror,* March 21, 1996.

181   *"from under a hundred to several million":* Liam Donaldson's estimate was made in urging the British government not to lift a ban on selling beef on the bone. "What is absolutely clear," he added, "is that the present relatively low number of cases of CJD should not lead anyone to conclude that the worst is over." James Hardy, "CJD Could Still Kill Millions, Says Prof," *The Mirror* (London), September 22, 1999.

181   *Tests of the appendices:* The tonsil and appendix study was reported in "Prevalence of Lymphoreticular Prion Protein Accumulation in UK Tissue Samples" in *Journal of Pathology,* Vol. 203(3), July 2004, pp. 733–39. Preliminary results had already prompted the government to commission a still ongoing study of the tonsils of 100,000 Britons.

182   *he pronounced the meeting:* Martin Enserik, "After the Crisis: More Questions About Prions," *Science,* Vol. 310 (5755) (December 16, 2005), pp. 1756–58.

182 *Among the most puzzling:* Clare's story was recounted by her father to the BSE Inquiry in March 1998 while she was still alive.

184 *"Did you look":* "Mad Cows and Englishmen," first broadcast on BBC 2 on February 15, 1998.

184 *"We were the experts . . .":* Ibid.

185 *crossed into a goat:* This news came in the form of an announcement by the European Commission on October 27, 2004. The goat had been chosen at random as part of a surveillance program. Tissue from the animal was then injected into mice and caused the symptoms of mad cow.

CHAPTER 12: **THE WORLD ACCORDING TO PRIONS**

187 *"I go to bed":* quoted in Antonio Regalado, "U.S. Research Into Prion Diseases Is Limited," *Wall Street Journal,* January 2, 2004.

187 *space dust:* The suggestion was first put forward by the distinguished astronomer Sir Fred Hoyle, who believed British cattle then picked up bacteria the dust contained. "In our opinion it was the nearly unique English practise of out-wintering cattle that explains why BSE hit English farms more severely than elsewhere," Sir Fred wrote in a letter he co-authored with Chandra Wickramasinghe to the *Independent* in 2000. More allegorical is this posting written by T. Chase on a New Age website: "Mad-Cow Disease infecting people's brains was announced on March 20 1996 in England as the Comet Hyakutake passed by the constellation. . . . Virgo the Virgin. I think that virgo the Virgin represents Isis, the Egyptian Goddess portrayed with cow's horns, giving us a 'cow' connection. And Virgo may also represent Europa, representing Europe, who rides a bull, again giving us a 'cow' connection. And Europa on a bull sounds like the woman in the Bible's last chapter, the Book of Revelation, Revelation 17 named 'Babylon' who rides the beast of the Antichrist described in Revelation 13. . . . I think the woman is Europe. This woman Babylon has a cup in her hand full of filthiness, and the world drinks from her filthy cup. I think the filthiness in Europa's cup is Mad Cow Disease exported to the world by improper cattle raising practices." Posted at http://www.revelation13.net/BSE.html.

188 *"parkinsonism, Huntington's chorea, multiple sclerosis":* Kuru, Gajdusek to Smadel, August 6, 1957.

189 *Eldepryl:* M. Sano, et al., "A Controlled Trial of Selegiline, Alpha-tocopherol, or Both as Treatment for Alzheimer's Disease," *New England Journal of Medicine,* 336(17) (April 24, 1997), pp. 1216-22.

189 *indistinguishable from Huntington's:* "Huntington disease phenocopy is a familial prion disease," *American Journal of Human Genetics,* 69(6) (December 2001), pp. 1385-88.

191 *"astounding":* "Substance Tied to Alzheimer's in Coast Study," Lawrence K. Altman, *The New York Times,* December 7, 1983.

191 *"red hair":* Matt Clark with Deborah Witherspoon, "A New Clue in Alzheimer's," *Newsweek* (December 19, 1983).

192 *"essentially indestructible":* Christopher Dobson, a protein biologist at Oxford University, "The Mechanism of Amyloid Formation and Its Link to Human Disease and Biological Evolution," in A. Agelli, et al., *Self-Assembling Peptide Systems in Biology, Medicine and Engineering* (Dordecht, Boston: Kluwer, 2001), p. 69.

192 *the disease can even be transmitted orally:* Per Westermark et al., "Transmissibility of Systemic Amyloidosis by a Prion-Like Mechanism," *Proceedings of the National Academy of Sciences,* 99(10) (May 14, 2002), pp. 6979-84.

192 *transmitted Alzheimer plaques in 1993:* "Evidence for the Experimental Transmission of Cerebral Beta-amyloidosis to Primates," *International Journal of Experimental Pathology,* 74(5) (October 1993), pp. 441-54. Some researchers ask whether Ridley and Baker's results were contaminated by prions in their lab.

192 *George Glenner, Prusiner's collaborator:* Rudolph E. Tanzi made the comment to me. See also Tanzi and Ann B. Parson, *Decoding Darkness* (New York: Perseus, 2000), p. 132.

193 *"the great tragedy of science":* Wöhler in a letter to his former teacher Joens Jacob Berzelius. Berzelius's prescient response was that if you could make urine, why not semen? "What masterful art to make such a tiny child in the laboratory of the technical school," he wrote.

193 *"chemical processes dependent upon common chemical forces":* quoted in Brock, *Liebig,* p. 205.

194 *The prion researcher Byron Caughey:* "The Chemistry of Scrapie Infection: Implications of the 'Ice 9' Metaphor," *Chemistry and Biology* (January 1995), pp. 1-5.

194 *"No hotel could offer"*: Gajdusek, *Jail Journal* (May 4, 1997); *"at the rate I am going:* Ibid (March 2, 1997). Gajdusek did not print this journal in the quantity of his previous published ones; in fact, there are only eight copies of the book in the world's libraries.

194 *"a great Buddha"*: unpublished interview. Courtesy of Robert Draper.

195 *"He wishes to roll"*: quoted in "Out of prison, Gajdusek Heads for Europe," *Science,* Vol. 280, no. 5364 (May 1, 1998), p. 663.

195 *"a 'virus' from the inorganic world"*: D. Carleton Gajdusek, "Molecular Casting of Infectious Amyloids, Inorganic and Organic Replication: Nucleation, Conformational Change and Self-Assembly," in A. Agelli, *Self-Assembling Peptide Systems,* p. 110.

196 *"We have had the Stone Age"*: Gareth Cook, "No Assembly Required for These Tiny Machines," *Boston Globe,* October 16, 2001.

CHAPTER 13: **DID MAN EAT MAN?**

198 *"European plagiarism"*: W. Arens, *The Man-Eating Myth* (New York: Oxford University Press, 1979), p. 84.

198 *early Highland patrol reports:* For example, John McArthur wrote in patrol report #1, Goroka subdistrict, 1952–53, p. 23: "It was firmly established by the members of [a previous patrol] that the people of the Wamu valley were cannibals." And similarly, regarding a famous incident during World War II, he wrote to district headquarters, "The Reverend Goldhardt informs me that . . . about 1944, a party of Australian soldiers found that the survivors of a Liberator aircraft crash had been killed and eaten. I have no record of this here. Have you anything on file?" (Patrol report #6, Goroka subdistrict, 1952–53, p. 2).

198 *"If opportunity presents itself"*: Skinner, patrol report #5, Kainantu subdistrict, 1947–48, p. 8.

199 *John Collinge undertook:* His key paper is "Balancing Selection at the Prion Protein Gene Consistent with Prehistoric Kurulike Epidemics," *Science,* 300 (5619) (April 25, 2003), pp. 640–43.

202 *Elio Lugaresi and Pierluigi Gambetti:* "Clinical Features of Fatal Familial Insomnia: Phenotypic Variability in Relation to a Polymorphism at Codon 129 of the Prion Protein Gene," *Brain Pathology,* 8(3) (July 1998), pp. 515–20.

203 *They died mostly from accidents:* For my summary of Stone Age health, a field known as paleopathology, I have relied on various texts, including Tony Waldron's *Shadows in the Soil* (South Carolina: Arcadia, 2001), Chapter 5, "What Did Our Remote Ancestors Die Of?"

205 *an important archaeological site:* A good introduction to Atapuerca can be found in a book by its co-director of excavations, Juan Luis Arsuaga: *The Neanderthal's Necklace* (New York: Four Walls Eight Windows, 2002).

206 *The official Atapuerca website:* www.ucm.es/info/paleo/ata/english/ sites/y-dolina/h-dolina.htm.

CHAPTER 14: **COMING TO AMERICA?**

210 *"a 90-year-old woman":* quoted in "Inquest Uncertainty over CJD Death," BBC News, April 27, 1991.

212 *American ranchers had imported:* Yam, *Pathological Protein,* pp. 153, 159.

215 *double its profits:* per the Motley Fool website, which calculated that Tyson Food would add more than $400 million to its bottom line if the ban on American beef were dropped (www.fool.com, May 19, 2005).

215 *The case of the Kansas beef producer:* Creekstone Farms sued the USDA in March 2006 to force the company to let it test all its cows.

216 *In the first study:* Richard Marsh, "Transmissible mink encephalopathy," *Revue scientifique et technique* (International Office of Epizootics), *Rev Sci Tech,* Vol. 11 (2), (June 1992), pp. 539–50.

216 *actually died of CJD:* Elias and Laura Manuelidis, "Suggested Links Between Different Types of Dementias: Creutzfeldt-Jakob Disease, Alzheimer Disease, and Retroviral CNS Infections," *Alzheimer Disease and Associated Disorders 3* (1989), pp. 100–109.

217 *"The laboratory folks":* Donald G. McNeil, Jr., and Alexei Barrionuevo, "For Months, Agriculture Department Delayed Announcing Result of Mad Cow Test," *The New York Times,* June 26, 2005.

218 *to its horror:* Eiji Hirose, "Johanns claims downer cattle did not have BSE," *Yomiuri Shimbun,* February 19, 2006.

220 *letter to the FDA:* The letter was written by a government relations vice president at McDonald's. "We are most concerned that the FDA has chosen to include a provision that would allow tissues from deadstock into the feed chain," the executive wrote. "We do not support the provision to

allow the removal of brain and spinal cord from down and deadstock over 30 months of age for several reasons. . . . Firstly, there are two issues regarding the complex logistics of this option. We do not feel that it is possible to have adequate removal especially during the warmer months. In addition, we do not feel that there are adequate means to enforce complete removal. Unlike slaughterhouses, there are no government inspectors at rendering plants or deadstock collection points" (December 19, 2005).

220 *David Asher:* In 1999, for instance, Asher told an interagency panel set up to monitor America's CJD risk that he didn't "believe that the issue [of sporadic CJD] is settled at all."

221 *"Why Vicky?":* "Infected Meat Linked to Dying Girl; Victoria Rimmer," *The Times* (London), January 26, 1994.

221 *"I couldn't see bloody Satan":* The speaker was the brother-in-law of Jean Wake, the meat-pie worker whose mother John Major had lectured to that humans could not contract mad cow disease.

225 *"Antlers—there is something magical":* from the website for Quality Deer Management, www.qdma.com/articles/details.asp?id=21.

225 *"We'd come from dairy farming families":* Mike Irwin, "CWD: Report from Ground Zero," *The Capital Times* (Madison), July 20, 2002.

226 *"ardent hunters":* Mary Van de Kamp Nohl, "The Killer Among Us," *Milwaukee Magazine* (December 2002).

227 *"Eradication is a nice idea":* quoted in "Chronic Wasting Disease Still Should Be a Priority," *Green Bay Press-Gazette,* July 14, 2005.

227 *a "national emergency":* When the USDA called CWD a "national emergency" it also quickly added that the term was just a semantic necessity for the transfer of new funds to CWD surveillance. "[It] does not mean that the United States is facing an extraordinary animal disease event," the agency pointed out in a press release, wary, as all government agencies are, of the Internet and the speed at which information travels.

227 *the "threat-from-within":* Aguzzi made his comments at the Days of Molecular Medicine conference in La Jolla, California, in March 2002; they were reported in "TSE threat to US Increases," *Nature Medicine,* Vol. 8 (5) (May 2002), p. 431.

231 *tiny amount of BSE:* Lasémzas, et al., "Risk of Oral Infection with Bovine Spongiform Encephalopathy Agent in Primates," *Lancet,* February 26–March 4, 2005, 365(9461), pp. 781–83.

231 *It better fits the model:* When I wrote these words, which were first published in *The New York Times Magazine* in 2004, I had not thought of the
possibility, later put forward by Colm Kelleher, that the restaurant equipment itself might have been contaminated (*Brain Trust* [New York: Pocket
Books, 2004], p. 190). While not impossible, such a cluster still seems to
me very unlikely. No doubt hundreds of premises in England were contaminated in this way, yet few clusters were identified and none proven.

232 *The longest odds of all:* D. Carleton Gajdusek, "Creutzfeldt-Jakob Disease
in a Husband and Wife," *Neurology,* Vol. 50 (3) (March), pp. 684–88. See
also an earlier paper of Gajdusek's in *Transmissible Subacute Spongiform
Encephalopathies: Prion Diseases,* L. Court, B. Dodet, eds. (Paris: Else-
vier, 1996), pp. 433–44. Gajdusek believes the couple were infected by an
unknown route.

232 *"Absence of evidence":* The remark is usually attributed to the British astronomer Martin Rees, but he told me he did not originate it.

232 *avid gardeners:* Gibbs made these comments on *Dateline,* March 14, 1997.
They are more significant than they might seem, since Gibbs was a clear-
inghouse for CJD cases at the NIH for decades.

233 *"I have had problems":* The posts appeared on CJD on www.CJDVoice.org
on the following dates: "Weird spells," August 26, 2004; a supplement for
breast enlargement, September 2, 2004 and November 16, 2004; "the
fact that you're not only alive," June 17, 2005; "the foil hat crowd," June
26, 2005; "Quitt offering false hopes," February 18, 2006; "at the moment, what else is there?," February 23, 2006.

CHAPTER 15: **FOR THE VICTIMS OF FATAL FAMILIAL INSOMNIA**

240 *only three pharmaceutical companies showed up:* "At Long Last, Signs of a
BSE Breakthrough: We May Soon Know the Size of the CJD Epidemic and
How to Treat It," *The Guardian,* September 5, 2001, p. 16.

241 *got the credit:* The two papers in order of appearance are Doh-Ura's "Lyso-
somotropic Agents and Cysteine Protease Inhibitors Inhibit Scrapie-
Associated Prion Protein Accumulation," *Journal of Virology,* Vol. 74 (10)
(May 2000), pp. 4894–97, and Prusiner's lab's "Acridine and Phenoth-
iazine Derivatives as Pharmacotherapeutics for Prion Disease," in *Proceedings of the National Academy of Sciences of the United States of
America,* Vol. 98 (17) (August 14, 2001), pp. 9836–41.

242 *another father with a sick child:* I draw the details of the Simms case from Lisa Belkin, "Why Is Jonathan Simms Still Alive?" *The New York Times Magazine* (May 11, 2003), as well as interviews with Donald Simms.

244 *"the worst case of abuse":* The O'Reilly Factor, December 5, 2003.

245 *thirty patients:* The source for these numbers is the CJD Alliance.

AFTERWORD: **A NOTE ON THE AUTHOR**

250 *It is a hodgepodge:* Although Charcot-Marie-Tooth disease is the most common hereditary neuropathy, it is so little known that one researcher recalled getting a grant to study CMT with the notation "Your request for research on tooth decay has been approved." (Recounted in "Researchers Lupski & Chance Study a Baffling Genetic Disease—Their Own," in *Journal of the American Medical Association,* Vol. 270 [19] [November 17, 1993], pp. 2374-75.)

252 *"the silence of the organs":* quoted in David B. Morris, *Illness and Culture* (Berkeley: University of California Press, 1998), p. 52.

252 *Charcot, the great French neurologist:* quoted in Rudy Capildeo, "Charcot in the 80s," from W. Clifford Rose and W. S. Bynum, eds., *Historical Aspects of the Neurosciences* (New York: Raven Press, 1982). I have often wished I could meet Charcot and beat him for his condescending rapture.

254 *"the greatest compliment you can make":* quoted in Christopher G. Goetz, *Charcot the Clinician: The Tuesday Lessons* (New York: Raven Press, 1987), p. 175.

254 *"a small fortune":* The story is told in *Collected Papers by Sigmund Freud* (New York, London: The International Psycho-analytical Press, 1924), Vol. 1, p. 13.

256 *"The prognosis is deplorable":* The story appears in Goetz, *Charcot,* pp. 171-74.

INDEX

Page numbers beginning with 261 refer to endnotes.

ABOUT THE AUTHOR

D. T. MAX was born and raised in New York City. His essays, reviews, and re-
porting on literature, culture, and science have appeared in *The New Yorker,*
The New York Times Magazine, Los Angeles Times, The Wall Street Journal, San
Francisco Chronicle, and *Chicago Tribune.* His work has been anthologized in
The Best American Science Writing 2006 and elsewhere. He lives outside of
Washington, D.C., with his wife, two children, and a rescued beagle who came
to them also named Max.

ABOUT THE TYPE

This book was set in Bodoni Book, a typeface named after Giambattista Bodoni, an Italian printer and type designer of the late eighteenth and early nineteenth century. It is not actually one of Bodoni's fonts but a modern version based on his style and manner and is distinguished by a marked contrast between the thick and thin elements of the letters.